TONY WALTER

WHAT DEATH MEANS NOW

Thinking critically about dying and grieving

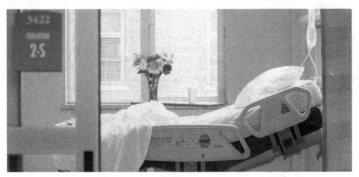

POLICY PRESS SHORTS INSIGHTS

First published in Great Britain in 2017 by

Policy Press
University of Bristol
1-9 Old Park Hill
Bristol
BS2 8BB
UK
t: +44 (0)117 954 5940
pp-info@bristol.ac.uk
www.policypress.co.uk

North America office:
Policy Press
c/o The University of Chicago Press
1427 East 60th Street
Chicago, IL 60637, USA
t: +1 773 702 7700
f: +1 773 702 9756
sales@press.uchicago.edu
www.press.uchicago.edu

© Policy Press 2017

British Library Cataloguing in Publication Data
A catalogue record for this book is available from the British Library.

Library of Congress Cataloging-in-Publication Data
A catalog record for this book has been requested.

ISBN 978-1-4473-3736-2 (paperback)
ISBN 978-1-4473-3751-5 (ePub)
ISBN 978-1-4473-3752-2 (Mobi)
ISBN 978-1-4473-3741-6 (ePDF)

Cover design by Policy Press
Front cover: image kindly supplied by Getty

Contents

Notes on author

Tony Walter works with the University of Bath's Centre for Death & Society where he is Honorary Professor. A sociologist, he has researched, written and taught about death and society for 30 years; before that, he wrote on a range of topics including religion, landscape, social security reform and basic income. His 15 books include *Funerals – and how to improve them* (Hodder, 1990), *The revival of death* (Routledge, 1994), and *On bereavement: the culture of grief* (Open University Press, 1999); co-edited books include *Pilgrimage in popular culture* (Macmillan, 1993) and *Social death* (Routledge, 2016).

Acknowledgements

My appreciative thanks to Klaus Wegleitner for commenting on a draft, and to the staff at Policy Press for the collaborative way they work with authors. The scholars who over 30 years have inspired me to think analytically and critically about death, dying and bereavement are too numerous to name; they too have made this book a collaborative product. The past decade working in the Department of Social and Policy Sciences at the University of Bath has encouraged me to consider policy issues more directly. Finally, I thank family, friends and neighbours who continue to teach me what dying and caring are like these days.

Acknowledgements

Introduction

What death means now

Though death comes to all humans, the challenges it poses evolve. This book outlines the particular challenges death poses today and how individuals, families, communities and societies are responding. The focus is on advanced industrial societies, especially those western countries that privilege individual autonomy – a resource that can be peculiarly compromised by bodily decline and by the uncertainties of dying, funerals and grieving.

Thinking critically

Death's contemporary challenges have prompted a raft of what, drawing on the sociological concept of moral entrepreneur, might be termed '**death entrepreneurs**' – individuals and movements promoting new and, in their view, psychologically healthier and more natural ways to die, funeralise and grieve. In North America, such entrepreneurs have collectively been labelled the **death awareness movement**; in the UK, they are represented by **palliative care**, **bereavement care**, the **compassionate community** movement and organisations such as *Dying Matters* and the *Natural Death Centre*. Death entrepreneurs typically urge us to take control of our deaths, to make choices, to express our feelings and to de-medicalise death.

Their prescriptions (like my own approach to university teaching) have been driven more by passion, belief and hard-won experience than by careful evaluation of the evidence. Thus, in the UK advance care planning is promoted, good hospice care is claimed to reduce requests for euthanasia, parents are advised to hold their stillborn baby, and mourners are advised to express their grief – even though evidence is either absent or queries such practices and claims. Halpern (2015, 2001) recently observed that 'no current policy or practice designed to improve care for millions of dying Americans is backed by a fraction of the evidence that the Food and Drug Administration would require to approve even a relatively innocuous drug'. This book, rather than signing up uncritically to the tenets of the death awareness movement, aims to promote critical thinking – to be a loyal critic of the movement.

The book's perspective

The perception of time as linear, a perception privileged in modern western societies, implies two narratives of history – a progress narrative and a decline/nostalgia narrative (Zerubavel, 2003). These two narratives dominate thinking about death and dying. In the progress narrative, medicine and public health have made and continue to make great strides in preventing and curing disease and extending longevity. In the decline narrative, modern medicine's view of the body as a machine to be fixed is inappropriate at the end of life and denies the dying person's humanity, while the erosion of community and religion undermine ritual, leaving us rudderless as we face the existential challenges of dying, grief and sorrow. Two of the most influential books in the field – by Swiss American psychiatrist Elisabeth Kübler-Ross (1969) on dying, and by English anthropologist Geoffrey Gorer (1965) on grief – start with a nostalgic account of a death from the author's childhood that they contrast with the mid-twentieth century's inhumane deathways. In each book, the author's decline narrative comprises a clarion call for change.

Though there are grains of truth in each, this book adopts neither the progress nor the decline narrative. Social, economic, religious and demographic changes often have an impact on the human experience of death and loss, and now is one such time. Societies often struggle to adapt their death practices to new circumstances, and there was no golden age when every member of society faced death and loss with equanimity; nor will there be. Humans and their societies endeavour to meet the Grim Reaper as best as they can.

Though my perspective is broadly sociological, I draw on work from many other disciplines. Interdisciplinarity is necessary not least because, as André Gide wrote, 'Death is always a struggle between what is rational, and what is not rational' (quoted in Rotar, 2015,145). The rural Greek villagers studied by anthropologist Loring Danforth (1982) understood the post-mortem fate of body and soul in profoundly symbolic ways, while at the same time – as farmers – knowing full well that 'when you're dead, you're dead'. Even sophisticated urbanites may not be immune from contradiction and irrationality, for example choosing a grave where the deceased will enjoy a good view or be sheltered by a tree (Francis et al, 2005). On departing from the sociable warmth of a post-burial wake one chilly January, I caught sight of my deceased friend's grave-mound through the churchyard fog and felt for her: cold, isolated and alone in the ground; here was I, an agnostic with a doctorate in sociology, imputing feeling to a corpse. Both before and after death, rational policies and practices must take into account the power of feelings (which may or may not reflect neat stage theories) and beliefs (which may or may not reflect formal religious teachings).

What the book is not about

The book focuses on the kind of death readers are themselves most likely to face – the everyday peacetime deaths, often in old age, that characterise economically developed, western countries. In order to highlight western assumptions, occasional contrasts are made with Japan. The book omits:

• tragic but relatively unusual deaths such as deaths of babies, road traffic accidents and disaster;

- threats to life at a societal or global level (for example, inequality, war, global warming) that can be tackled only through major political change;
- death in low to middle income countries – even though these comprise the majority of deaths today;
- euthanasia and assisted suicide;
- intentional or unintentional killing by professionals (notably soldiers, doctors and veterinary surgeons) through war, abortion, medical error, medical euthanasia, battlefield euthanasia, or the euthanising of animals;
- killing by non-professionals, whether through accident (not least on the road), or murder/manslaughter;
- suicide;
- scientific, medical or educational use of human remains through archaeological excavation, museum display, dissection or organ donation;
- the sometimes extensive and long-term effects of disaster (such as the Black Death, or Chernobyl).

Each of these omissions deserves a book of its own.

Outline of the book

Chapter One assesses conflicting understandings of why death is not always handled as well as it might be in modern western societies. Some see the problem as wrong ideas about death, while others point to healthcare systems that become unfit for purpose as death approaches. Chapter Two interrogates the idea that it is good for people to talk about death and dying.

The following chapters progress from dying through to funerals, disposing of the body and grief. Chapter Three critiques the contemporary western 'good death' in which the person continues for as long as possible as an autonomous individual able to make choices, remaining in control as far as possible, and accompanied by others. Given how frequently death's medicalisation is criticised, Chapter Four explores different views of the role of healthcare professionals at the end of life, and the 'compassionate community' approach that aims to de-professionalise dying and return it to families and communities with medical expertise as servant rather than master. Chapter Five discusses evolving understandings of the purpose of the funeral as societies become more affluent and, often, more secular. Chapter Six examines the ongoing challenge of disposing of very large numbers of bodies in contemporary mega-cities in ways that respect emotional sensitivities, religious diversity, physical hygiene and ecological sustainability. Chapter Seven analyses evolving norms about 'healthy' grief.

In a world in which many people are geographically separated from those they love yet are digitally connected, Chapter Eight explores migration and digital communication in relation to dying bodies and graves that are largely or wholly immovable. Finally, the conclusion identifies a new paradigm – pervasive death – that is emerging not only intentionally from the activities of the death awareness movement but also unintentionally through digital communication.

ONE

What's the problem?

Demographics make death and dying a global twenty-first century issue. Many western societies experienced a post-war baby boom, which will lead to a dying boom from 2020 to 2050. Much of the global South will see an even bigger dying boom as an unprecedented number of babies survived the latter half of the twentieth century to grow up, age and eventually – in the twenty-first century – die. David Clark and colleagues (2017) estimate that global annual deaths, currently around 56 million, will reach an all-time high of around 90 million by the middle of the twenty-first century before going down later in the century – reflecting fertility rates that over the past four decades have been declining throughout the world outside sub-Saharan Africa. Managing dying, dead bodies and grief is therefore a major twenty-first century issue – for individuals, for families, for communities and for social and health policies around the world.

Who dies and of what is changing. In the global North, and increasingly in the global South, death is moving from the province of infancy and childhood, to that of old age. In England and Wales in 1900, 25 per cent of deaths were of infants under a year old; by the end of the century, this had fallen to only 1 per cent of deaths. In 1900, only 12 per cent of deaths were among the over 75s; within a century this had increased to 59 per cent of all deaths (Davies, 2015,

21). Similar patterns are found in almost all industrial societies, with few exceptions. Poorer people, however, have higher death rates at all ages and from almost all diseases, the differences between the highest and lowest social classes being particularly marked, and increasing, in the UK (Fitzpatrick and Chandola, 2000; Dorling, 2013).

Clean water, efficient sewers, secure supply of food and reduced family size greatly reduce death from infectious disease, a trend evident in the UK from the 1870s; inoculation and, from the mid twentieth century, antibiotics also help, though to what extent has been debated (McKeown, 1979). With infants and the elderly particularly vulnerable to infections, most people in the global North and increasing numbers in the South now live through to old age where they become vulnerable to conditions that develop with age. Chronic, non-communicable disease now accounts for almost two thirds of all deaths in the world, and 80 per cent of such deaths occur in low and middle income countries. Cancer exemplifies this, as does the degeneration of various organs – heart, lung, brain, kidneys, etc – often in combination. Tuberculosis excepted, dying from infectious disease often took just a few days or a week or two, whereas dying from the conditions of older age often entails months or years of frailty, illness, multiple medications and procedures, and reduced functioning. This period entails considerable costs – not only for formal health and social care (however paid for), but also for family carers who may lose earnings or bear other costs including their own health. The World Health Organisation states that 'the exorbitant costs of non-communicable diseases are now forcing 100 million people into poverty annually, stifling development'.[1]

Prolonged dying may be sketched in terms of **dying trajectories** (Figure 1.1). i) Only around one death in ten is **sudden**. ii) In **terminal illness** such as cancer, functioning can often be maintained for months or years before a rapid decline a few weeks before the end. iii) **Organ failure** comprises a series of episodes (such as heart attack or stroke) each of which, though not fatal, reduces subsequent functioning until the final fatal episode. Living with such a condition, or conditions, can last years or decades, often with considerably reduced functioning, lowering quality of life and morale. iv) Frailty 'is the fragility of multiple body systems as their customary reserves diminish with age and disease' (Lynn and Adamson, 2003, 5). Often including dementia, it entails '**prolonged dwindling**'; with few reserves, small setbacks easily escalate. Trajectories ii), iii) and iv) each account for around 30 per cent of those who die in contemporary western societies. In trajectories iii) and iv), predicting when death will come is not at all easy. In most western countries, the proportion of people dying on trajectory (ii) (cancer) is going down, while those dying on trajectory (iv) (frailty) is going up.

Figure 1.1: Dying trajectories

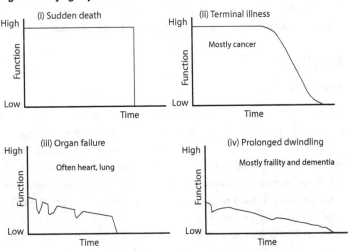

Source: adapted from Lynn and Adamson, 2003, 8
Copyright holder: RAND Corporation, Santa Monica, CA. Reprinted with permission.

Traditional religious end of life rites – in the European Middle Ages termed the *ars moriendi* or art of dying – were developed at a time when death typically came a few days after falling ill. In those few days, the person made peace with their family and their God. Today, by contrast, humans typically live for months, years or even decades with a disease or diseases that may or will eventually kill them, requiring what Lofland (1978) has called **a new craft of dying** – which arguably is what the death awareness movement and palliative care offer (Walter, 1994). This new craft, however, has been developed largely with people dying of cancer whose terminal phase is relatively predictable, who usually retain full cognitive capacity until the last day or two and who therefore retain considerable agency. Developing a craft that works for those on trajectories iii) and iv), especially where dementia is involved, is still a work in progress.

This chapter looks at two widely disseminated kinds of claim about what is wrong with contemporary western societies' response to this new landscape of death and dying. One claims we have our ideas about death all wrong. The other claims that social structures and organisational systems make contemporary dying particularly hard.

Wrong ideas?

Unfamiliarity

Through human history, most children learnt about death by growing up in a one-room dwelling where they witnessed siblings or a parent die over a few days from infection. But, starting in the global North in the late nineteenth century and now almost everywhere outside sub-Saharan Africa, learning about death through direct observation has, mercifully, ceased to be a normal part of growing up, though a class differential remains. The actual moment of death is most likely to be in hospital or some other institution, with few or no family members present to witness it. Also, today's varied and often complex dying trajectories make it hard for families to apply lessons from one death to the next, which in any case may not occur for some decades. As French historian Philippe Ariès (1981) puts it, modern people are largely **unfamiliar** with death. They have therefore handed knowledge about dying over to healthcare professionals. In sociological language, death has been **medicalised** (Kellehear, 2016) and **sequestered** from everyday life (Mellor and Shilling, 1993; Bayatrizi and Tehrani, 2017).

So how do people today learn about death and dying? On occasion, learning still occurs in the family when grandparents or pets die. Otherwise, modern humans learn through the mass media about the deaths of strangers, celebrities and fictional characters depicted in soap operas, movies, music, art and literature from the Harry Potter novels to auto/biographies about dying and bereavement; news media are disproportionately about death, though not the kinds of deaths audiences are likely themselves to face (McIlwain, 2005; Kitch and Hume, 2008; Coombs, 2014). Such images can create unrealistic and often overly negative assumptions about what dying is like (Kellehear, 2014). More interactively, digital natives who grow up with social media now encounter a range of deaths of those who are neither intimates nor complete strangers when, for example, their Facebook friends post messages about or to a deceased grandparent or other intimate; digital natives have developed new online codes of condolence for when friends of friends die (Walter et al, 2011–12). It is therefore now hard to reach adulthood unaware that people die or without having posted an online condolence. What is lacking, however, is first-hand knowledge of what happens physically to a dying or dead body, the spiritual pain of dying, caring for a dying family member, how to arrange a funeral, or the searing pain of grief. We can only be thankful that most twenty-first century children are spared such experiences, but it does leave today's citizens with a legacy of ignorance about death, sometimes lasting until late middle age when eventually one's own parents die.

Taboo

The ignorance of many modern people about death and dying is indisputable. What *is* disputable is the frequent claim that death is **taboo** in contemporary western society. Certainly some individuals, some families, and some work or leisure groups may shut down conversation about dying and grief, or feel uncomfortable about it, while Chapter Two discusses two very specific kinds of death that *are* surrounded by taboos (sometimes imposed by the very people claiming to bust all death taboos). And in the next section, I note that those close to a dying person are often less willing to talk about what is happening than is the person him- or herself. But there is little evidence of a society-wide death taboo in the west – witness the various media representations of death and loss mentioned in the previous paragraph. Death sells newspapers, books, movies, by the bucket load; far from marginal, it is integral to the capitalist economy of western media. Or consider higher education: the social science modules on death that I and colleagues teach may be seen as different and interesting by students, but neither I nor to the best of my knowledge my colleagues have ever been sanctioned for breaking a taboo. Chinese culture may be different, where in the New Year period it is unacceptable to dwell upon death or indeed anything negative which could bring bad luck.

Denial

If the existence or non-existence of a social taboo should be fairly easy to spot, another claim, that death is **denied** – denial being one of several unconscious defence mechanisms identified by Freud – is much more problematic to verify or falsify. Some individuals may deny their own mortality, but a more complex argument is that societies in general, or modern society in particular, is death denying. Extending unconscious defence mechanisms from individual to society is problematic (Kellehear, 1984) yet has proved an enduringly popular idea ever since the publication in 1973 of cultural anthropologist Ernest Becker's book *The Denial of Death*. Becker presumed three things: first, humans are terrified of their own mortality; second, this terror is so terrifying it has to be repressed; third, this repression of death profoundly shapes culture, politics, morality and many other aspects of social life.

Becker argued that repression of mortality – more even than (as Freud suggested) repression of sexuality – drives both individual personality and civilisation in damaging ways. He put it thus (p 53), 'The irony of man's condition is that the deepest need is to be free of the anxiety of death and annihilation; but it is life itself which awakens it, and so we must shrink from being fully alive.' Without religion's illusory comfort, death anxiety is deemed to wreak particular havoc in modern secular societies. Becker's thesis gave rise 15 years later to **Terror Management Theory** (TMT), which has subsequently been tested in over 500 social psychology experiments around the world, demonstrating that the more people are reminded of their mortality the more, for example, they protect their self-esteem by embracing cultural values such as nationalism and prejudice against outgroups. Sociologist Zygmunt Bauman (1992) also drew on Becker to argue that humans deal with their awareness of finitude and death by constructing culture.

A more limited version of Becker's theory is that, though awareness of finitude is universal, this does not universally cause terror; terror becomes prevalent in certain social or psychological conditions. Thus Mellor and Shilling (1993, 414), drawing on sociologists Peter Berger and Anthony Giddens, suggest that in late modernity 'The more people prioritise issues relating to self-identity and the body, the more difficult it will be for them to cope with the idea of the self ceasing to exist.' Gunaratnam (2013) argues that the terrors experienced by elderly migrants may build on cumulative experiences of loss, abuse, oppression over one or more lifetimes. Malcolm Johnson (2016) observes how some older people fear their own end because of an unfulfilled life. All these authors acknowledge fear of one's own death – not as universal but as arising from particular social or personal conditions. A life cycle perspective might add that fear of one's own non-being can be particularly marked in adolescence, but much less so in a contented old age.

Talcott Parsons, by contrast, argued that twentieth-century America directly confronted human mortality and managed it in the only way it knew: rationally and pragmatically through practices such as life insurance and public health (Parsons and Lidz, 1963). Some decades later, Phil Zuckerman (2008) argued that those living in what he considers the world's most secular society – Denmark – rather than being terrified of death without the support of religion, in fact face it with remarkable equanimity.[2]

Other scholars point to death of the other rather than of self as the typically modern anxiety. Ariès (1981) argued that different epochs in Western European history have been characterised by different paradigms of death – what he called *mentalités*. Dominating the late Middle Ages and the Renaissance was fear of *my* death – what will become of me when I die? In the nineteenth century, however, the Romantic movement emphasised a different concern, *thy* death – if the meaning of life is love (of partner, of child), then what will become of me when *you* die? Today, after the long and healthy lives many enjoy, being dead is little to be feared – yet unprecedented longevity has deepened ties with close family and friends, making their loss the greater anxiety (Blauner, 1966). Poll almost any group of westerners today about what they most fear about death, and losing an intimate will trump fear of one's own death. And when people are coming to the end of their life, it is more often those around them who may be unwilling to acknowledge the impending departure. Such evidence questions how universal is fear of my own death, suggesting instead the dominance today of fear of death of the other (Walter, 2017).

Psychological **attachment theory** suggests a more universal significance of loss of the other. Though children come in due course to realise their own mortality, experiencing loss of the other comes far earlier: the infant's greatest terror is experiencing its mother's (it does not realise, temporary) absence. Some psychoanalysts consider that the infant experiences this as death of self, but the unadorned fact is that sheer terror at the other's absence precedes any conscious anticipation of one's own extinction. The infant's manifest primal fear is not of its own non-existence, but of the mother's absence, which in healthy childrearing is managed by secure attachment to a mother figure. Unfortunately, TMT experiments focus on awareness of death of self, not death of the other.

Overall, Becker's ambition to link the personal, the social and the political is impressive, but he uses too heavyweight a theory – denial – to explain what can often be more easily explained in terms of unfamiliarity. This, along with the health that many enjoy for decades, means that for many people for much of the time death is not so much denied as out of sight and therefore out of mind. Though some individuals may deny their mortality, many more write a will, take out life insurance, and get on with living. This does not amount to a society that denies death.

It may, however, allow false or superficial values to dominate. And here the evidence is mixed. On the one hand, there are many reports of people who find that a life-threatening illness in mid-life or a near death experience (NDE) causes them to re-visit their values and to re-focus on what they consider really important to life; if they survive, they may change career, divorce or move home in order to live more authentically (Kellehear, 1996). Living in the light of mortality is surely no bad thing, as Psalm 90 acknowledged three millennia ago: 'Number our days, that our hearts may incline to wisdom.' On the other hand, the 'life-reviews' that many Americans conduct in old age typically assure them that their life (marriage, family, career) was good enough, enabling them to continue into life's last phase with equanimity (Butler, 1963); in the UK, life-centred funerals typically assure mourners that the deceased's life was more than just 'good enough' (Walter, 2016b). Death awareness can thus either challenge or validate a person's participation in the consumerist rat race.

Be that as it may, the death awareness movement has inherited the assumptions of the 1960s' counter culture that taboos are there to be broken; that denial and repression are bad; and that feelings should be acknowledged. Who cares, therefore, about evidence for death denial and repression; the mantra that death is denied gives the movement a liberatory aura, as Lynn Lofland astutely noticed back in 1978. Chapter Two explores this further.

Wrong structures?

The other common critique of dying in the modern west points to the social structures and organisational systems in which the dying find themselves (Sudnow, 1967; Foucault, 1973; Illich, 1976; Kaufman, 2005). As Lofland (1978, 83) put it, extended dying means that 'for many contemporary humans, goodly portions of their dying time is spent in hospitals, under the control of medical practices and beliefs and regulated by the rationalised concerns of medical bureaucracies. Proponents and sympathizers (of the death awareness movement) have not found these arrangements satisfactory.' A number of issues have been identified.

Religion and community

It is often thought that death was handled better in pre-industrial times. The argument usually has two components. First, when people lived in small-scale communities, not only could the dying person – having already witnessed others die of the same infection – recognise the signs of their own dying, but they found themselves dying at home within a known community. True, death often came before old age, and the dying did not have access to modern pain relief, but they were not isolated and marginalised. They were not shunted off to hospital, nor was their home invaded by dozens of strange professionals. Second, religion is presumed to have provided a framework for belief and/ or ritual action that gave meaning to death. Today, by contrast, the deathbed is characterised by ignorance, a struggle to make sense of things ('Why me? I've enjoyed only a couple of years of retirement!'), and anomie – a sense of normlessness and uncertainty as to what to do.

It is easy to romanticise death in past times. Personally, I would rather die a twenty-first century hospital death as a frail 93-year-old, than an eighteenth-century home death from cholera aged 13. And the evidence that secularisation makes death and loss harder is not clear cut. A strong belief or philosophy, whether religious or atheistic, seems to serve the dying and grieving well; what makes things hard is the *process* of secularisation, lasting a generation or two, as older people lose their childhood faith and churches no longer provide the support older people may still expect (Coleman et al, 2015). More serious is how dying people today find themselves surrounded by strangers in unfamiliar surroundings – the care home, the hospital – where their prime status is not that of grandmother or sister but of patient.

Healthcare

Healthcare systems around the world vary in their organisation and funding but most are struggling in one way or another. In the USA, the multiplicity of providers and insurers generates considerable administration costs and undermines service co-ordination, while the much-reduced service available to poorer Americans leads to poor national healthcare outcomes, all at greater expense than in comparable countries (Lynn and Adamson, 2003). Fear of litigation may lead to heroic but futile treatment that is not only expensive but also damages quality of life as it nears its end (Kaufman, 2005). In the UK by contrast, the **National Health Service** (NHS) is poorly funded compared to healthcare in comparable countries, and suffers from frequent politically driven reforms.

Given that a significant proportion of healthcare expenditure goes on the last year of life (Aldridge and Kelley, 2015), strains on the system bear disproportionately on those nearing death. Healthcare demands will grow further as the baby boomers near the end of their lives, while the working population who pay – whether through taxes or insurance contributions – declines in proportion. Already in the UK, social care of the frail elderly – whether in care homes or their own home – is inadequately resourced, creating extra pressure on healthcare. Unsurprisingly, recent years have witnessed several scandals concerning care of Britons nearing the end of life. I will mention just two. From 2005 to 2008, managerial targets and economic/political pressures at the Mid Staffordshire hospital permeated working practices, radically reducing the time staff had to do personal care; hundreds of vulnerable patients, mainly those who were elderly, died prematurely after suffering terrible standards of 'care' (Francis, 2013). In 2011, Southern Cross, operator of 752 care homes, became insolvent, raising questions about the private sector's ability to provide consistent and reliable residential eldercare (Scourfield, 2012; Lloyd et al, 2014). At the same time, though palliative care in the UK has been judged to be the best in the world (EIU, 2015), it benefits only a minority of dying Britons; good palliative care for those dying of cancer does not solve the resource issues or structural strains that underlie the end of life care scandals affecting frail elderly Britons.

Abstract systems

A deeper critique claims that healthcare institutions, however well-resourced and structured, are inevitably large, complex bureaucracies which neither those who work in them nor patients and families fully understand (Kaufman, 2005). This means that, however competent and caring its personnel, their decisions may reflect (often hidden) organisational constraints more than patient need. The person facing their own unique end finds him- or herself caught up in an organisational system that is more complex and impenetrable than any they have hitherto encountered (Walter, 1994). As Fong (2017) argues, three powerful institutions – medicine, the market, and the media – frame contemporary understandings of death and dying.

Medicalisation

Perhaps the most common 'system' critique is that medicine, geared to curing disease, does not provide the best frame for thinking about death or the best context for managing dying (Illich, 1976; Bauman, 1992). If most past cultures personified death, for example as 'the Grim Reaper', modern medicine deconstructs it into hundreds of medical conditions; family members as well as healthcare professionals resort to medical accounts, for example when well-wishers ask how the dying person is. Kellehear (2016) argues that medicalisation not only places dying people within inappropriate systems and organisations, but also fosters wrong ideas, which he calls myths. One myth is the seduction of medical rescue; when hope of cure fades and dying is eventually recognised, other medical rescues swing into action: palliative medicine, euthanising medicine (in certain countries), acute care medicine and care homes. Dying becomes a medical event, rather than a natural event in which medicine plays a part (see Chapter Four).

Medicalisation continues after death. Modern cemetery and crematorium designs are dictated more by public health and environmental safety than by religious requirements – protecting the health of the living is now more important than assisting the soul's journey. And then in the ensuing months and years, bereavement is to an extent medicalised. People struggling with bereavement are more likely to consult a doctor than another professional, while bereavement research and the development of bereavement care have been substantially shaped by psychiatry – a medical specialty. Disposing of bodies and mourning have become health issues.

The critique of dying's medicalisation has recently led to an alternative proposal, that dying should be seen primarily as a social and community responsibility. Just as **the social model of disability** proposes that people are disabled more by how society treats them than by their physical or cognitive condition, so the compassionate community approach to dying seeks to integrate dying (and bereaved) people within their communities, without reverting to nostalgic ideas about 'community'. This approach, like the critique of medicalisation, links wrong systems with wrong ideas; it is examined in Chapter Four.

Questions

How would you assess the various diagnoses of what is wrong with death and dying in advanced industrial societies? Are there factors not identified in this chapter?

Notes

[1] www.who.int/features/factfiles/health_inequities/facts/en/index4.html

[2] Kjaersgaard Markussen (2013) argues that how Danes deal with death is not as irreligious as Zuckerman supposes.

TWO

Good to talk?

Dying matters – let's talk about it.
(Strapline of the UK Dying Matters Coalition)

Those who identify the problem as death being unfamiliar, taboo or denied – the 'wrong ideas' camp identified in Chapter One – often see the main solution as talk. Talking about what had hitherto been taboo will, they believe, enable individuals to:

- have better deaths because they can prepare themselves, their family and their doctor for what they want at the end of life;
- in the meantime, live more authentically in light of their mortality;
- possibly even save society from racism, materialism and other social evils caused by society's supposed denial of death.

This 'talk' agenda has long characterised the death awareness movement, and finds its latest incarnations in Britain's Department of Health-funded **Dying Matters Coalition**, and globally in the fast-growing **death café** movement – where urban strangers meet each other over coffee and cake for an hour or two to talk about death.

This chapter takes a more sober look at the benefits of talking about death and dying – whether in a healthcare setting, within the family, in a death café, or in some other context. First I set out some good reasons to talk; then some questionable reasons to talk; and, finally, the limits of what talking can achieve.

Good reasons to talk

A very good reason for individuals, families, communities or an entire society to talk about death is that what death means is changing. Throughout most of the world, humans are living longer and often dying in different ways from their parents, grandparents and great-grandparents. As infections came to cause fewer deaths, cancer became, in mid-twentieth century western countries, public enemy and private fear number one; in the twenty-first century, a lingering dying from or with dementia is perhaps becoming an equal fear and challenge. After death, as formal religion weakens in many western countries, traditional funerals make little sense to increasing numbers of mourners, while across the entire world social media are changing how mourners interact with each other. Talking with interested and/ or knowledgeable others is part of exploring how to live and die in this evolving landscape.

Given that I may not expect the death nor want the funeral my forebears had, there is merit in expressing any preferences I may have about the end of my life. As we will see shortly, there is no guarantee such preferences will be actualised, but there is considerable evidence that discussing and clarifying preferences, whether with family or healthcare professionals, can enhance a sense of control.

Though North American and northern European doctors have become much more open with patients about a terminal cancer diagnosis than was the case in the mid-twentieth century (Novack, 1979), this openness has yet to extend to other major killers such as heart disease, circulatory disease and dementia, perhaps because the likely timing of death is much less clear. In countries where the individual is expected to take charge of his or her own destiny, there is evidence that greater openness by healthcare professionals can enable patients and families to make better informed decisions about how to live and about care. In those many countries, for example in Eastern and Southern Europe and in Asia, where sick individuals are expected to defer to doctor and family, the pros and cons of doctors telling the full story to terminal patients rather than to their family are less clear (Maruyama, 1997).

With death publicly framed by medicine, by the media and by commerce, some baby boomers, expecting to exercise control over their lives, may feel it liberating to reclaim their own understandings of death – for example through talking in death cafés, or through taking control of actual practices, whether that be assisted suicide or disposing of the body (Fong, 2017).

Talking about personal fears of death and dying, both in advance and when the time comes, can be helpful, especially if people are willing to listen when the person wants to talk. As the end approaches, talking enables family and friends to say goodbye, which if not done might be later regretted and add to the sorrow of bereavement. Intimates who do not want to acknowledge an impending death can contribute to the dying person's loneliness; open acknowledgement, by contrast, can lead to greater intimacy (Elias, 1985). What is not helpful is pressure to talk about such an intimate matter when one or more parties are not ready or willing.

Questionable reasons to talk

It is often claimed that talking and stating preferences in advance of falling terminally ill are crucial if people are to have a good death. One local initiative to encourage its local community to consider and explore end-of-life issues states that 'A lack of conversation is perhaps the most important reason why people's wishes go ignored or unfulfilled.'[1] However, the evidence for this claim is limited and what evidence there is, is mixed. Though some studies show that documented end-of-life plans reduce unwanted hospital admissions and enable more people to die in their preferred place, others show no effect, not least because of the organisational and financial constraints under which healthcare organisations operate – structures frequently trump individual agency (Kaufman, 2005). Even if the system requires patients to make choices, this is typically only at certain times and only certain choices are available (Kaufman, 2005), which could account for the mixed evidence – for it to be recorded and acted upon, you have to make your preference clear at the required time, to the required person. The care setting may also make a difference: end-of-life care plans made by hospice patients with cancer have a greater chance of being carried out than plans made by or for the frail elderly who are in and out of hospital as one crisis (such as pneumonia) succeeds another (such as a fall).

More dramatic is the claim that confronting and talking about mortality will save western civilisation. Jon Underwood, founder of the death café movement in the UK, has suggested[2] – reflecting Terror Management Theory (see Chapter One) – that consumer society is driven by the illusion that we will live forever; thus death denial drives capitalism. Talking about death at death cafés will therefore help create a more sustainable society. That talking for 90 minutes with a few strangers whom one may never meet again provides a short cut to economic revolution, the end of capitalism even, may be a heart-warming idea, but is a remarkably big claim.

The moral entrepreneurs who encourage everyone to talk about death make much of breaking a taboo. This ritual denunciation of taboo plays at least three functions. First, it implies that, were it not for the taboo, everyone naturally would speak about death and dying (Armstrong, 1987). It's not just that people *ought* to speak, but that it's *natural* to speak. Second, in some settings and voluntary organisations, this ritual denunciation binds together those who see themselves as brave enough to break the taboo – there's a feel-good factor. Third, with the death taboo identified as the enemy, those joining together to break it see themselves engaged in a moral crusade (Lofland, 1978). Given the lack of evidence for a society-wide death taboo (Chapter One), not to mention regular denunciations of this supposed taboo since at least the 1960s, one has to conclude with sociologist Lofland that the identification of a death taboo has to be understood not as social science but as rhetoric that motivates action, specifically the imperative to talk. As a reason to talk about death, taboo-busting is psychologically effective but objectively questionable. A better reason to talk is the first one listed in this chapter – what death means now is not what it meant a generation or two ago, so humans need together to develop new crafts of dying and mourning.

It may be that some who choose to talk about death, for example to strangers in a death café or in a blog, do so because there *are* death taboos in their own family or friendship groups. Whether talking to strangers, offline or online, actually helps people talk to their family, friends or to key healthcare personnel, however, has not been researched. It is possible that attendance at a death-awareness group may do the opposite, confirming the participants' desire to talk and alienating them further from their family. We simply do not know.

Limits to talk

National laws and identity politics in certain western countries make it very difficult to talk about two kinds of death – euthanasia (in countries where it is illegal) and regretted abortions (in countries with social media savvy religious lobbies, such as the USA). If there is no general social taboo on talking about death in modern society, there are some specific taboos in certain countries.

Euthanasia

American anthropologist Frances Norwood (2009) conducted a valuable ethnography in which she attended Dutch GPs' home visits to dying patients. She found that in the Netherlands euthanasia is more often a process of talking than of killing. Of the terminally ill who initiate and continue a conversation with their doctor about wanting euthanasia if things get too bad, only a small minority actually go through with it. And among those who are not terminally ill, talking to friends, family and doctors about the circumstances in which one might wish for euthanasia is a normal part of conversation in the Netherlands; it provides Dutch people with a language for talking about their values, standards, loves and loyalties.

The contrast with the UK could not be more striking. A Dutch doctoral student who came to my university to research elderly Britons' feelings about home as they neared the end of life was surprised to find how talking about when to die, taken for granted in Dutch society, rarely if ever occurred in her conversations with elderly Britons. She herself came to feel awkward talking about something which she had taken for granted before coming to Britain (Visser, 2017, 8–9). More formally, palliative care professionals and initiatives such as *Dying Matters* encourage people to talk to their family and doctor about *where* they want to die, and dying in the documented 'preferred place of care' is increasingly used as an index of a good death. These initiatives do not encourage people to talk about *when* they want to die, as this raises the issue of euthanasia, which in the UK is illegal. So some of the very initiatives that pride themselves on taboo-busting, collude with and even help solidify a very real taboo. Whether the UK should legalise euthanasia is often a matter for informal and media debate, but healthcare professionals steer individuals away from considering euthanasia as part of personally coming to terms with mortality or planning their last days.

Abortion

Another kind of death which some have good reason to keep quiet about is abortion, especially the regretted abortion. In the USA where abortion has become a powerful symbol in religious identity politics, there are two major discourses about abortion: that it is a woman's right to choose, and that in taking a life it is a sin. The first rarely acknowledges that some who chose an abortion in good faith may come subsequently to regret it and to suffer deeply. This is reflected in social science research, where the emotional costs of miscarriage, stillbirth and infant loss have been widely researched and highlighted, but any emotional costs associated with abortion, however rare (Lee, 2003), are ignored. The second discourse invites those who have aborted to confess and find God's forgiveness. The woman who regrets an abortion but cannot embrace the Christian discourse therefore has nowhere to turn – the pro-choice movement does not want to hear, the pro-life movement offers an answer she finds unhelpful. These American discourses have now gone global on the internet and in English language social media, so the polarisation of American abortion politics now has an impact on women in other countries who seek help online.

In Japan, by contrast, a rite for aborted foetuses, *mizuko kuyō*, has developed since the 1970s (LaFleur, 1992; Klass and Heath, 1997). In a society where apologising often initiates a social encounter, the rite allows the mother to apologise to the foetus. The entrance path to many Buddhist temples are now lined by rows of baby statues, each paid for by one or both of the parents. As well as apology, their motivations could include grief, comforting the foetus' soul, guilt, or fear of retribution from the foetus's spirit. The wider context is a society in which there are shrines apologising to foxes, working animals, tailors' needles – anything that has been destroyed or discarded (Kretchmer, 2000). The *mizuko*, the water child, is understood within this tradition. Abortion in Japan is not politicised.

Other limits

A very different limit to talk is the uncertainty for most people of how and when they will die. Though I know that sooner or later I will be dead, as a 68-year-old in good health I have very little idea of how or when I will die; nor do I know what my family or other circumstances will be at the time. Curiously, it is thus much easier to talk in an informed way about being dead than about dying. In its 2013 campaign, *Dying Matters* invited Britons to do five things: 'Write a will; record your funeral wishes; plan your future care and support; consider registering as an organ donor; and tell your loved ones your wishes.' Significantly, three of these (wills, funerals, organ donation) concern what other people should do after your death, one is very general, and only one concerns end-of-life care. Similarly, death café conversations frequently include discussion of funerals, including home funerals, ecological burial and funeral poverty (Fong, 2017).

That it is okay to talk about death is a good message. But this does not mean that everyone needs to talk about death all the time. Some people will not want to talk about it, or certain aspects of it, now, in this group, with this family member or with this healthcare professional. And they should not be criticised for not wanting to talk. Many military veterans do not talk about their wartime experiences to family members whose comprehension of active service is necessarily limited, but they may value playing pool every Friday night at the veterans' club – not talking about death, loss and trauma, simply being in the company of others who comprehend. One small study of Holocaust survivors found that those able to adjust to post-war life not only did not talk about their camp experiences, they did not even dream about them; while not forgetting their experiences, they 'avoided, both in wakefulness and in sleep, the recurrent penetration of the feelings... they had felt during their confinement' (Kaminer and Lavie, 1993, 345). Repression can be a highly effective defence mechanism.

Questions

Is it good to talk about death? When might it not be?

Notes

[1] www.finity.org.uk

[2] At a meeting at the Camden Collective, London, 24 September 2013.

THREE

A better way to die?

The space between reality and expectation is a hard place to exist.
And choice? Real or imagined? Helpful or burdensome?
(Kevin Bolster, palliative care physician)

Chapter One sketched how the pattern of dying changes as societies
develop economically. Dying from infection over a few days gives way
to people living with their, or a family member's, cancer, dementia,
heart or lung disease for years – a period which allows for a new kind
of living as well as of dying. In response, a new craft of dying (Lofland,
1978) – or to be more precise, a new craft of living-dying – has been
developed, especially in English-speaking countries.

This new craft is rooted in three things. First, the hospice and
palliative care movement's experience of working with people dying
of cancer, a disease with a relatively clear trajectory that rarely impairs
cognitive capacity; second, baby boomer values, including the freedom
to choose one's own life; third, neoliberal political ideology, especially
as manifested in healthcare. Each of these presume an individual agent,
willing and able to make informed choices about his or her life. Out
of this mix has coalesced a new craft of dying, characterised by open
communication, choice, control and a natural, accompanied death –

echoing, at the other end of life, new crafts of birthing. Promoted by palliative care, baby boomers and neoliberal healthcare, how relevant is this craft to the majority of those dying today – in old age and with conditions other than cancer? This chapter offers a critical assessment.

The new craft of dying

Communication, autonomy and choice

Since the mid-twentieth century, medical ethics and practice have become less paternalistic, valuing the principle of patient autonomy more highly in relation to medical beneficence (Verkerk, 1999). If following doctor's orders was the old mantra, neoliberal medicine requires open communication enabling a partnership in which the doctor's expertise invites, indeed requires, patients to make choices about treatment and symptom management. In this new regime, patients are required to make informed choices, not least as they approach the end of life (GMC, 2010) – despite a lack of clear evidence that this is what people want. Dutch philosopher and ethnographer Annemarie Mol (2008, 97) observes that when 'patients complain about bad healthcare, they may mention that they were not given a choice, but more often they talk about neglect'. This is also found in the UK where healthcare scandals at end of life concern not lack of choice but lack of care. Yet neoliberalism continues to promote informed choice along with individual responsibility for and self-management of health, not least at the end of life (Seymour et al, 2005; Conway, 2011). So even as our bodies are falling apart, we are enjoined to be self-determining consumers, agents rather than patients, doing rather than being done to, whether or not that is what we want.

This image of good dying is expressed in the healthcare practice of **advance care planning** (ACP), in which doctor and patient (or, if lacking mental capacity, the family) discuss future care. Enabling people to live their last days and months as they would want is an aim of hospice and palliative care. In many countries, the individual's right to be master or mistress of their own dying is key to the argument for legalising euthanasia – something that many palliative care practitioners and some terminally ill people reject. It is very different from notions of good dying traditionally found in Mediterranean and East Asian societies in which the dying person defers to family and doctor.

Teresa Maruyama (1997) sees hospice's promotion of individual autonomy as rooted not in neoliberal ideology, but in the Christian concept of the pilgrim, a link made explicit by hospice founder Cicely Saunders who used the word 'hospice' to link to medieval hospitality for pilgrims. The dying person becomes a pilgrim, walking their personal path to redemption, very different from the Japanese transformation of the dying person into a 'baby' to be looked after by doctor and family – a role encouraged by Japanese culture's valuing of dependence.

Sharon Kaufman, who conducted an insightful ethnography of dying in an American hospital, focuses less on neoliberal ideology or cultural history than on an institutional requirement to solve problems and make decisions. Hospital language 'redirects incoherence, anxiety, breakdown, diffuse suffering, and any other expression of affect that lacks rationality' into 'control', 'choice', 'the good death' – neat, abstract concepts that assume individual autonomy (Kaufman, 2005, 17).

Of course, coma, stroke or advanced dementia may turn the person into a baby more than a pilgrim, or at any rate not the ideal autonomous agent capable of ticking a hospital bureaucracy's neat boxes. The remedy currently being promoted is that everyone in good health should make clear their end of life care preferences long before they become unable to express such preferences. In the UK, for example, the 2005 **Mental Capacity Act** recognises three ways to prepare for mental incapacity. First, if I wish to state specific wishes in advance, such as no life support if in a coma, I can make an **Advance Directive** (AD). Second, a **Lasting Power of Attorney** (LPA) gives control over care and/or finances to a specified friend or family member should I become mentally incapacitated. Or third, I can make no advance provision and leave care decisions when mentally incapacitated to a **best interest decision** by doctors at the time.

ADs and LPAs are common in the USA; research into their effectiveness has been of variable quality and thrown up divergent findings, though there is evidence of an increase in patients' chances of receiving the kind and level of care they would want (Silveira et al, 2010). In the UK, rather few ADs and LPAs have been made to date and questions have been raised about their effectiveness. ADs need to be immediately available to any who might act on them, such as ambulance crew or emergency room personnel – unlikely unless tattooed on the chest. ADs based on forms available on the internet can too easily be worded in ways that are unclear or not legally binding. People may make a financial LPA and mistakenly think it covers care as well. And when there is no AD or LPA, some doctors think that 'best interest' equals clinical judgement rather than taking into account the patient's values as described by family or friends.

Control

Some argue that a sense of control is more important than choice. In her studies of later life, British researcher Anne Bowling found that 'feelings of little or no control over their lives also statistically increased people's risk – by over three times – of rating their quality of life as bad rather than good, compared with those who felt they had a lot to some control'. Both ACP and euthanasia conversations can enhance the sense of control. The ACP process may give the person reassurance that things will be under control, even if events later render the plan redundant. Likewise, being able to talk about euthanasia provides Dutch people with a sense of control over their life should suffering become intolerable, which Norwood (2009) suggests reflects Dutch society's long history of having to control nature if the country is not to disappear under water.

An anecdote illustrates the importance of the sense of control. Over several months, a seriously ill elderly friend saw 12 doctors in four hospitals until her condition was identified, and identified as terminal. Her experience of fragmented care, lack of diagnosis, lack of a single professional in charge of her care, and arguably a lack of compassion, all led this hitherto self-determining retired academic to feel powerless, scared and depressed. Contra those who argue against the medicalisation of dying, her experience of the medical system's *lack* of control of her case was what caused her to feel powerless. This was not resolved by giving her more choices, still less by avoiding medical care, but – eventually – by one palliative care physician taking control and coordinating care. Her depression lifted within a day or two. Patient choice therefore needs to be complemented by coordinated, effective systems – though as Kaufman (2005) reminds us, bureaucratic systems have a life of their own.

Natural dying, holistic care

The new craft sees dying as a natural event. Medicine can play a role in managing pain and symptoms, but ultimately dying – like giving birth – is a natural, human process. The hospice movement therefore promotes holistic, multi-disciplinary care, in which the patient is re-conceived from a sick body to a whole person with emotional, psychological, social and spiritual needs as well as – and interacting with – physical needs. The deathbed is re-humanised, though as several sociologists have pointed out, this is less the process of de-medicalisation that its proponents sometimes imagine, and more one of further medical colonisation with the palliative care team now empowered to peer into not only the patient's body but also her very soul (Arney and Bergen, 1984; Rose, 1989; Clark, 1999).

Accompanied

Finally, healthcare professionals and some family members see the good death as accompanied – people should not take their last breath alone. Kellehear (2009), however, suggests that some old people living and dying alone may be exercising agency by resisting attention from their family or from formal services. Caswell and O'Connor (2015) identify a contradiction between the accompanied ideal and the ideal of dying at home. Since many elderly people live on their own, and choose so to do, dying at home may well entail dying alone and may be what some want. So far, however, dying alone has been little researched; it has much more often simply been asserted as bad.

Communication, choice, control and an accompanied natural death are promoted in policy and in healthcare practice, not least palliative care. I will now enquire how these values interact with and are constrained by inscrutable systems, failing bodies and contrary values.

A constrained craft

Unresponsive systems

Though promoting choice at the end of life is part of healthcare policy in most English-speaking countries, choosing euthanasia is not a choice that healthcare professionals can assist in jurisdictions where it is illegal. Clearly, systems offer some choices and not others.

In so far as choices for end of life care *are* offered by healthcare practitioners, they depend on practitioners identifying that the person is dying and discussing this with the person and their family. Unfortunately, dying is often seen by practitioners as a bodily condition of the final few days or even hours, rather than a social role a person may adopt for months or years, so choices are often offered and made very late (Kellehear, 2016).

What choices can be made then depends on resources – the family's, the community's and the healthcare system's. If the person or their family cannot afford the care they desire, for example full-time care at home, then they will only be able to access what care the system offers, such as part-time care, or a care home. Where care is not freely available to all, as with healthcare in the USA or social care in England and Wales, a two-tier system can constrain poorer people's choices.

Even when well resourced, healthcare systems are complex, bureaucratic and – increasingly – profit seeking. Kaufman demonstrated how American hospital staff are caught between organisational structures and demands on the one hand, and the needs of suffering patients and families on the other. Likewise in the UK, without coordination of services, choice means little (Seymour et al, 2005). Even within one service, system needs may trump personal needs, as illustrated by agencies providing home care for people with dementia, a life limiting disease. Because of underfunding of care agencies and the complexities of organising rotas, people living at home with dementia may host a cavalcade of different carers coming in several times a day, even though they need the same few carers they can recognise and get to trust. While UK policy encourages a dementia-friendly society, the organisation and resourcing of home care for people with dementia militates against this.

To be informed, choices about care by people facing the end of life and by their families need good information about the various care options. Which hospital or care home is best? Can we trust this home care agency's promise to provide consistency of carers? Previous experience may be partial and hence a poor guide. A bad experience in hospital may be followed next time by a much better experience in the same hospital but in another ward.

My own 91-year-old mother was deeply unhappy in the geriatric hospital in which she found herself after breaking her ankle; how were we, her children, to gauge the quality of care in various alternative hospitals? Our saviour turned out to be Alison, my mother's hairdresser who, specialising in older housebound clients, had continued to do their hair as they moved to hospital or care home. She immediately named for us three settings where our mother would be content, and we got her transferred within 36 hours. Unlike formal inspectors, Alison was an unthreatening secret observer of each of the institutions she visited, and proved for us a reliable guide.

How could Alison's role be made available to all families seeking similar information? Care settings for those nearing the end of life are, in terms of audit, like restaurants. Technical medical and nursing procedures, like a restaurant's kitchen, need inspecting by technical inspectors. But most end of life care is not technical, resembling instead a restaurant's ambience – best assessed by mystery shoppers who collectively author good food guides, or by more informal online ratings like TripAdvisor. Such assessments abandon the myth of objectivity embedded in overt inspection, and those perusing TripAdvisor ratings understand them to reflect subjective experiences to be taken on overall balance. To date, care agencies in the UK do not receive this kind of collective, honestly subjective, bottom-up online rating, so information about these agencies remains sparse at a time when comparable information about customer experience in restaurants, hotels and holidays expands exponentially. Despite the rhetoric of informed choice, it is hard for people nearing the end of life, or their families, to continue in the prescribed role of informed consumer.

Failing bodies

If information about care provision is limited, information about what I would feel should I become chronically or terminally ill and dependent on others is even more elusive. I might feel worse than is implied in the Christian idea of suffering as redemptive, though some who fear dependency have come to discover a new humanity in receiving. When physical self-maintenance – getting up, washing, going to the bathroom – takes not minutes but hours out of each day, hours leaving one exhausted to do anything else, does this change personal values which were honed in earlier life when physical vitality was taken for granted? Will the values of those baby boomers currently enjoying a third age of active retirement change when in time they come to experience the limitations of the fourth age in which agency begins to slip away (Lloyd, 2004)? They cannot know in advance, for frailty and dementia are – to use Gilleard and Higgs' striking analogy (2010) – black holes from which little or no 'light' emanates. Though there are many books, articles and blogs by cancer sufferers reporting their experiences, few frail elderly people or people with dementia report back from the front line, or at least not to society at large. How then can I know in advance what kind of life would be intolerable?

Research does indicate that frail old people typically take one day at a time. A recent British doctoral study found that

> Frail older people experience profound uncertainty, associated
> with rapid changes to their physical and/or mental state and

complex challenges in everyday life. Consequently, their attention is focused on day-to-day maintenance of quality of life, rather than on future care or advance decision making. Many had difficulty imagining a future...The end-of-life orientation of current ACP policy and practice is at odds with the dynamic nature of frailty...The liberal idea of autonomy as self-determination and self-interest presented by the legalistic and ideologically driven policy of ACP is out of step with the lived worlds of frail older people. (Bramley, 2016: ii-iii)

Bramley, like other critics, goes on to argue for a **relational ethic of care** (Verkerk, 2001; Lloyd, 2004; van Heijst, 2011), reflecting a feminist relational ethic in regard to all persons, sick or healthy (Gilligan, 1982; Tronto, 1994). Indeed, any good carer understands that care is a two-way relationship (Mol, 2008).

Consistent with this, research into advanced dementia indicates that a person's emotional life may remain considerably more intact than their linguistic and cognitive abilities, meaning that they can convey feeling and even ethical stances. Unfortunately, western societies tend to prioritise reason over emotion, and language over non-verbal expression. Advance care planning and advance directives prioritise reason and language, and trade on fears of their loss; this positions people with dementia as less fully human than is implied in a more relational and emotional understanding of human-ness (Boyle and Warren, 2017).

What, though, about comatose patients? An unpublished paper by the Japanese sociologist Hiroshi Yamazaki (2008) helps us think about this. He argues that western palliative medicine's script for the good death, in which open communication enables the patient to make autonomous choices, condemns to a bad death the dying patient with 'no apparent awareness of dying and (who) cannot make autonomous decisions' such as those in coma, after a major stroke, or with advanced dementia. Western commentators often do indeed see this as a recipe for **social death**, in which the body lingers but the person has gone. Analysing one of Japan's many medical mangas

– cartoon stories which (like western medical soap operas) explore healthcare ethics and dilemmas – Yamazaki finds that the Japanese have a script for a good comatose death, for 'living as a comatose patient still involves interactions and exchanges with both formal and informal carers'. Throughout life, Japanese culture's relational self, though now undermined by western society's autonomous self, practices *omoiyari* – considering others through empathetic reading of their non-verbal behaviour; thus in this manga, nurses gauge empathetically 'unvoiced needs, providing comfort without actually being asked' (Yamazaki, 2008, 17).

Readers who, like myself, have received traditional Japanese hospitality may well have experienced being cared for without having to be asked what they want or need, which the Japanese call *amae*, the pleasurable state of depending on the benevolence or goodwill of others – a pleasure which Doi (1981) notes we first experience as a baby. Many western patients have experienced this too; it's just that, especially in neoliberal healthcare, we struggle to find a language for it. Drawing on Tronto's (1994) four elements of care – attentiveness, responsibility, competence and responsiveness – and refusing to restrict love to the private sphere, Dutch healthcare unions *do* have a term: **professional loving care** (van Heijst, 2011). But the English have a word for its opposite: feeling *abandoned*. Being abandoned and neglected is at the heart of many eldercare scandals, and feeling abandoned is the experience of many vulnerable patients as they get shunted around a complex healthcare system with, it seems, no one in charge of their case. Interestingly, in Japan where being looked after is so highly valued, stories abound of old people being abandoned (Danely, 2014); the worst evil to befall Japanese citizens toward the end of life is not lack of choice, but abandonment. If some western citizens feel likewise, end of life care strategies have yet to recognise it (Borgstrom and Walter, 2015).

Bodywork

Compatible with this is another diagnosis: the low status of those who wash, feed and toilet other people's disintegrating bodies (Twigg, 2006), especially in class-conscious Britain where those seeking professional status disdain manual labour. The nursing profession now delegates body care as far as possible to minimally trained care assistants whose intimate body work is not closely monitored by supervisors; in care homes, supervisors and inspectors rarely if ever peer into old people's nappies to check if they have been changed.[1] Recent care scandals in the UK have typically been about bodywork: food being left out of reach of care home residents or hospital patients, residents not helped to the toilet, patients not turned over in bed. Underpaid, understaffed and undervalued bodyworkers who care *about* residents and patients are often poorly resourced to care *for* them; workers may use their own time to provide extra care to make up for the system's deficiencies (Cohen, 2011). There is also the danger of undervalued bodyworkers with little control over their conditions of work taking it out on even more powerless residents/patients/clients. Properly resourcing and valuing bodywork is essential if the quality of dying is to improve.

Contrary values

The image of the dying person in control, making choices about how to live in the meantime, though increasingly influential in policy is not shared by all. The dying person may embrace or encounter other ideas and values.

Family conflict

Other ideas and values may be held by other members of the person's family. As my failing body and/or mind makes me depend more on – and quite possibly live in closer proximity to – family, conflicting values which once could be kept at arm's length may rub up against each other precisely when I am least able to stand my ground. Different interpretations of religion, differential trust in medicine versus alternative therapies, the conflicting needs of the dying person and those who will survive them, all can make dying harder than living, eroding the dying person's sense of control and capacity to make autonomous choices. Helping families with such issues is the stuff of palliative care social work.

Migration

Among the increasing numbers from the global South moving to work in the global North, those who do not return home will die in the North (Gunaratnam, 2013). As several studies have shown (Winzelberg, 2005), not all migrants share the North's passion for the autonomous individual – when it comes to decision making at the end of life, family can be more important than the individual, and religion more important than personal autonomy. And ideas of the good death may well differ. For some, such as Senegal's Wolof people, the bad death is a death abroad, outside the community (Evans et al, 2016). In a previous book (Walter, 1994), I outlined a trichotomy summarising how dying has changed, contrasting how authority in dying and mourning has shifted from family/religion, to medicine, to the individual (see Table 3.1).

Table 3.1: Authority and the good death

Society:	Traditional	Modern	Post/late-modern
Authority:	Family/religion	Medicine	Individual
The good death:	Within the community	Pain and symptoms controlled	Dying 'my way'

The kind of dying increasingly privileged in postmodern, neoliberal western health policy is thus culturally specific. But migrant experiences are far from homogenous. Though dying at home within one's community, surrounded by family and buried in one's own land is an extremely common construction of the good death around the world, members of migrant families who live between two worlds may not all agree on where home is or who counts as family and thus what counts as a good death (van der Pijl, 2016).

Religions

Religions often have specific requirements for how to die and mourn. British Hindus, for example, may wish to follow the requirement to die on the floor, surrounded by chanting relatives performing traditional rites. This may be challenging for hospitals, care homes and hospices to accommodate, despite policies that the dying person should have as much choice and control as possible, and be accompanied (Firth, 1997). Fundamentalist varieties of Christianity, Judaism and Islam see individual autonomy – the idea that people should be free to live and die as they wish rather than follow their Maker's revealed instructions – as an idolatrous manifestation of secular humanism. Thus fundamentalist Christians in the USA may oppose hospice care, or Orthodox Jewish women in Belgium may oppose euthanasia (Baeke et al, 2011). Within any one religion, there is typically as wide a spectrum of views of dying as of living.

Conclusion

This chapter has argued that currently fashionable policies for good end of life care that privilege patient choice and control are problematic and contested, both in principle and in many people's experience as they near the end of life. In conclusion, I suggest three other policy principles that should become more prominent.

Protection

After a lifetime of being reasonably protected by family, state, earnings and worldview, many members of affluent societies find themselves toward the end of life abandoned and unprotected – experiencing what Giorgio Agamben (1998) terms 'bare life' and Kellehear (2007) 'shameful death'. Protecting the vulnerable at the end of life with policies and practices comparable to those that protect children at the start of life should become a higher priority. Japan's *omoiyari* and *amae*, Tronto's care ethics, feminism's relational ethics and Dutch health workers' professional loving care all provide possible starting points, among others. And a policy that a person's care at the end of life should be overseen by one professional seems key to ending the sense of abandonment, though actually coordinating care within a fragmented system is easier said than done.

Preference

To choose implies that choice can be put into effect. Because of inscrutable institutions, failing bodies and contrary ideas, end of life choices often cannot be put into effect. But preferences can be expressed. To promise choices implies a degree of control that does not exist; to encourage the expression of preferences is more realistic, more honest. Unfortunately, the word 'preference' does not resonate so well with neoliberal politicians and healthcare managers, nor (in the English language) is it catchy in the way that 'choice' is – a one syllable synonym for 'preference' is sorely needed!

Enabling environments

The social model of disability, pointing to how social and physical environments disable, has been extended to dementia via the notion of the **dementia friendly society**. Since increasing numbers of people die of or with dementia, living as well as possible towards the end of life requires physical and social environments which are navigable by people with cognitive as well as physical impairments. Further ways that communities can be more friendly and compassionate for those facing the end of life with or without dementia are discussed in the next chapter.

These policies require a new kind of practice in which palliative care and eldercare become equal partners. For too long, eldercare has focused on active ageing, ignoring the final lap of frailty, dependence and death – though care homes have much experience of end of life. For too long, at least in the UK, palliative care has continued its founder Cicely Saunders' 'missionary' agenda of extending its British cancer-based expertise to every part of the globe and to every disease, rather than engaging in real dialogue with those who have extensive knowledge of dying with and from the conditions of old age and in other cultures. Committees tasked to develop end of life care policies for the UK continue to be dominated by palliative care, with token or no representation from eldercare. It is time to have a dialogue, to share power and influence, and to develop policy together.

Questions

What would you see as a good enough death in old age? What might prevent it from happening? What might make it more likely?

Note

[1]   My thanks to Jana Králová for this insight.

FOUR

What are professionals good at?

Death's medicalisation is contentious, yet doctors, nurses, ambulance crew and other health practitioners cannot but continue to act on the stage of contemporary western dying. What then should be their role in this particular drama?

The presence of health personnel on this stage is often highly valued. Technical competence in controlling pain and symptoms – at the heart of palliative care, geriatric medicine and general practice – is appreciated by family members as well as by dying people themselves. In the UK where healthcare is provided free at the point of access through the National Health Service (NHS), it can be a profound experience to feel cared for, looked after, taken seriously by people who know what they are doing, and all provided for free by the national community through taxation. Douglas Davies (2015) argues in his book *Mors Britannica* that the NHS, under whose varied ministry most Britons die, focuses national values of life and death at precisely the time when the established church has abandoned this role. I have witnessed this less in five-minute appointments with the GP than in ambulances and hospitals when life is at risk or coming to an end. In the hospital bed, and more especially within the ambulance, you are vulnerable yet in a total caring environment, like a womb. The English language may not have an equivalent for Japanese *amae* – the value of and pleasure in being looked after – but British people's passionate belief in and defence of their NHS represents an intuitive understanding of *amae*.

Since, however, Ivan Illich wrote *Medical Nemesis* (1975), death's medicalisation – especially within hospital where most people die – has been subjected to critique. Doctors are trained and hospitals designed to cure, so may not always be appropriate when someone is dying – a natural process that has no cure. Dying is a role and an identity (Kellehear, 2014) as well as a body breaking down, and **the dying role** does not entail **the sick role**'s 'contract' between doctor and patient (Field, 1996). What then is the health professional's role at the end of life? What should be the contract with the dying person and/or the family? I now consider the pros and cons of four professional roles – intervention, presence, enabling, and holistic care – before going on to examine the concept of compassionate communities which re-locates health professionals in a wider context.

Four professional roles

Intervention

The idea of the body as a machine and the doctor a mechanic with the skills and tools to fix it when it breaks down is based on a Cartesian mind–body dualism. The body can be detached from the rest of the person, and fixed. This formulation has been widely criticised, from both inside and outside medicine, not least at the end of life when the machine is irrevocably breaking down. At this point, the doctor-mechanic either abandons the broken machine – at precisely the point when its owner is facing one of life's deepest personal and existential crises – or the mechanic doctor continues to try to fix the machine long after such efforts become futile, often at great expense.

This critique risks caricature, so for a minute I would like to defend the doctor-mechanic. First, mechanics, whether patching up my car or my body, can do so with humour, skill and care. Second, I may wish to keep my existential crises to myself, needing the doctor simply for symptom or pain relief – even if s/he knows that physical pain can be influenced by existential pain. And third, though critics of medicalisation argue that humans are *more* than just a body, the lived experience of many fit and well people, not least in a Cartesian world that privileges mind over body, is to imagine ourselves as much *less* than a body. We tend to take our healthy body for granted, unaware of how it works, so to experience our broken body being paid full attention by someone who understands bodies may actually make us more, not less, whole people.

Even practitioners who reject Cartesian dualism often talk in mechanical language. Holistic practitioners increasingly talk in terms of **'interventions'**. Psycho-social initiatives to aid dying people, their carers, or mourners are often conceptualised as interventions, tested like drugs through controlled trials. Another revealing term is service 'delivery' – thus end of life care, like other services, is 'delivered' to patients and their families, as though care were a mail package. Indeed, we find talk of 'care packages'. Curious. People do not 'deliver' care to their own children or ailing parents, still less in 'packages'; rather, they care *for* them. Healthcare's translation of care, including holistic palliative care, from a verb to a noun implies its commodification: the turning of a human relationship into a discrete, limited, costable thing (Ungerson, 1997; Tronto, 2010). When healthcare workers do care for and about their clients, this is not because it is part of their paid-for, auditable labour but because – as one human encountering a vulnerable other human – they care (Cohen, 2011).

Presence

A very different understanding that sees care not as noun but as verb conceives the practitioner not so much, or not only, as one who intervenes in the patient's life but as one who is present with the patient. 'Watch with me' or attentive **presence** was central to how Cicely Saunders developed the practice of hospice care, and has subsequently been theorised by feminist ethicists and social scientists. Utriainen (2010), who describes presence with insight and clarity, considers it a form of active passivity, while (as we saw in Chapter

Three) care ethicists Tronto (1994) and van Heijst (2011) focus on its quality of attentiveness. They argue that the professional repertoire of intervention needs to be supplemented by presence, and the ethics of autonomy supplemented by a relational ethics of care. Love does not have to be restricted to the private sphere, to those with whom one is intimate or even to recipients who are conscious: people provide TLC (tender loving care) to buildings or gardens, so why not PLC (professional loving care) to vulnerable patients (van Heijst, 2011)?

Skilled interveners can be very present as they are intervening. The challenge is to professionalise presence so that it becomes part of the worker's professional identity, something which both the British hospice movement and Dutch healthcare unions have attempted, though the difficulty of measuring presence (Russ, 2005) remains its Achilles heel in 'the audit society' (Power, 1997). Randomised controlled trials can measure interventions; they cannot measure presence.

Enabling

Many palliative care workers see their role as helping or enabling patients to live as they want in their final weeks and to die as they want. Gunaratnam's (2013) book on migrants' experiences of palliative care in London is full of positive examples of nurses, social workers and other staff helping their patients and clients achieve the death they want in often quite difficult circumstances.

Holistic care

Palliative care aims to see the dying person not as a body to be fixed, but as a whole person with a potentially wide range of needs – emotional, spiritual and social as well as physical. Cicely Saunders' concept of '**total pain**' saw pain as multi-dimensional, with existential, biographical and physical pain inter-connected. The *doctor–patient* relationship is replaced by one in which the patient is surrounded by a multi-professional team

(Figure 4.1). Though the team typically includes a doctor, it need not be led by a doctor.

Figure 4.1 Palliative care multidisciplinary team

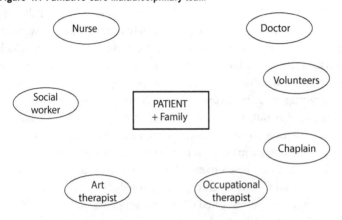

This all-embracing care can induce in families as well as patients a warm feeling of being looked after and is often deeply appreciated – reflected in the relative ease with which British hospices attract bequests from those they have helped and donations and volunteers from the local community.

This kind of total care, however, needs critical friends if it is not to drift into uncritical self-satisfaction. Those who pioneered it, such as Cicely Saunders in the UK (du Boulay, 1984) and Elisabeth Kübler-Ross in the USA (1969), were themselves doctors who – as we saw in the previous chapter – advocated an expansion of the medical gaze in which not only the person's body but also their feelings, relationships and worldview are potentially open to the doctor's scrutiny. Multi-professional palliative care teams, most of whose members are not doctors and many of whom wish to de-medicalise dying, end up expanding the *professional* gaze. In this hyper-professionalised dying, empowerment of the dying person and their family goes hand in hand with a certain disempowerment. This is illustrated by the many heartfelt post-death comments along the lines of 'I don't know how we'd have coped without those lovely folk from the hospice.' Humans have died for millennia without the assistance of multi-professional teams, but millions now depend on this kind of care. Is this, or is this not, progress?

Gender needs consideration here (Utriainen, 2010). Palliative care's founders were not only doctors, they were also mainly women. Throughout its 60-year history, holistic palliative care – in which physical sickness is linked to spiritual concerns, past hurts, the fear of dying, and so on – has been promoted significantly by women, contrasting with interventionist medicine's domination by men. Research has not, to my knowledge, investigated whether holistic care tends more to be appreciated by female patients and families; for example, do more males than females prefer their medical symptoms to be treated by a no-nonsense 'how do we manage this condition?' approach and to keep spiritual or emotional struggles to themselves? Nor has research investigated related dynamics within households, for example, how family members who prefer intervention from a medical 'mechanic' negotiate with other family members who see everything as connected and who value holistic care.

There are clearly also resource issues. High quality palliative care is labour intensive, and rolling it out beyond cancer to the longer and less predictable dying trajectory of frail old age would not be cheap. That said, palliative care is usually cheaper than heroic but futile surgical interventions.

Compassionate communities

The compassionate community concept applies takes the principles of the 1986 Ottawa Charter for Health Promotion[1] and applies them to end of life care which becomes a community responsibility – whether by 'community' we mean an entire city, a school or factory, or a dying person's own social network. Inspirations include first Kellehear's (2005; 2007) critique of palliative care's agenda (until very recently) to increase professional rather than community capacity. Second, both philosophically and practically, the compassionate community idea has much in common with the social model of disability and the dementia friendly society. Third, the Indian state of Kerala provides a large-scale and long-running model of how compassionate community can work at end of life. Local networks of 10 to 15 volunteers identify the chronically ill people in their neighbourhood, organise appropriate care and liaise with medical services; overall, the Kerala scheme covers a population of over 12 million people (Kumar, 2007).

Compassionate communities mobilise local social networks that do, or could, surround the dying person and their family carers. This can entail community development projects; volunteers, as in Kerala; or families mobilising their existing networks. A quick look at the burgeoning literature on support for family carers at end of life indicates how radical this idea is – almost all of this literature is about how *professionals* can support the carer, even though most support for carers comes from their existing informal social networks. The compassionate community model, by contrast, works with the grain of how humans normally support one another.

In this model, instead of a patient surrounded by a team of professionals in which family may just be visible but other social relationships are invisible or marginalised (Figure 4.1), we see the dying person and any informal carers at the centre of a social network including not only family, but also friends, neighbours, colleagues, employers, schools, faith community, and so on, with potential to help the person or more likely their carer with practical, social or emotional support (Figure 4.2). Inserted into this network are healthcare professionals with their own specific tasks (Abel et al, 2011). For actual examples of the social networks of people caring for a dying family member, see Leonard et al (2013) – crucially, their network 'maps' show the connections between everyone on the map, which for simplicity Figures 4.1 and 4.2 omit.

This reverses the classic palliative care model, which sees the community as marginal to professional care; instead, professional care plays various roles within a wider community of care. The doctor or nurse is just one among many actors on a community stage, rather than the community playing a bit-part on a medical stage. The more attenuated the naturally existing family or community networks, as can happen in extreme old age, the greater the likely role for volunteers or professionals. In other words, the less the dying person's **social capital**, the more formal care they may need. A key concept here is **network poverty**: 'The network poor are individuals who do not have the kind of social network configuration that is most appropriate for the stage of the life course they have reached, to enable them to thrive' (Perri 6, 1997, 27). Professional or volunteer assistance is therefore best targeted at the network poor. At present, it works the other way around: those with high social capital and good networks have the contacts to mobilise more professional care.

Figure 4.2: Compassionate community network

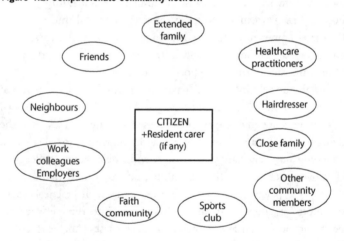

Two kinds of research are sorely needed to undergird compassionate community approaches to end of life care. First (Abel et al, 2011, 130), we need 'research evidence on how – in the absence of any professional encouragement to do so—families mobilise their social networks at the end of life.' Researchers disagree about the strength of existing communities and networks throughout life – witness the debate following Putnam's celebrated book *Bowling Alone* which claimed local social networks in the USA to be at an all-time low (Putnam, 2000; Fine, 2010). We do, however, know quite a bit about the social networks of the elderly (for example, Wenger, 1991; Gardner, 2011). Where these are robust, they lay a foundation for everyday compassion at end of life; but social networks can atrophy if an older person becomes housebound and/or develops dementia, rendering them vulnerable as they become more frail.[2] In the absence of knowledge about the extent to which families' existing social networks and community resources currently support end of life care, Abel et al (2011) ask whether compassionate community initiatives should focus on building capacity at the community level (for example, Kellehear, 2005) or on helping families mobilise their existing social networks as they care for a family member at the end of life (for example, Horsfall et al, 2011). One study (Walter, 1999a) found wide variation in neighbourliness from one street to the next, so solutions will not be one-size-fits-all.

Second, there need to be more evaluations of the effectiveness of the (as yet) rather few compassionate community projects (Wegleitner et al, 2015), though evaluations so far are encouraging (Sallnow et al., 2016). We do know that risk averse 'service delivery' organisations and systems resist coordinating with grassroots action taken by people acting not as professional or volunteer but as friend or neighbour, even if practitioners on the ground know of such friends and neighbours and their value (Horsfall et al, 2013). With friends and neighbours communicating with each other via social media, and healthcare organisations' IT systems firewalled against non-professionals, a fluid flow of information between professionals and carers seems unlikely. Kerala's integration of neighbourhood volunteers with formal healthcare is unlikely in most western contexts.

None of this has stopped compassionate community moving centre stage in end of life policy-making in some countries, including recently the UK. As with more conventional palliative care, passion not evidence is the original driving force. And as with more conventional palliative care (and some other areas of medicine), passion-driven initiatives will hopefully in time receive proper evaluation. Participatory action research has an affinity with community development, so will also have a role to play (Heimerl and Wegleitner, 2013).

Doing and talking

Compassionate community initiatives invite people to do as well as talk.[3] Here we should consider two views about how to promote change in health-related behaviour (Abel et al, 2011). One (favoured by community development approaches) is that breaking the so-called death taboo will enable people to talk about death and thus change their attitudes and actions (Chapter Two). The other view (favoured by approaches that mobilise families' existing networks) is that getting people involved in supporting other local people facing the end of life will change attitudes. The evidence from other public health initiatives such as smoking cessation and environmental initiatives such as household recycling is that attitudes can change behaviour, but also that behaviour can change attitudes: preventing people from smoking in buildings or requiring them to recycle forces behaviour change which in turn can change attitudes. Here is a hypothetical example of how this might work at end of life. A teenage girl offers to walk a dying neighbour's dog after school each day. Each time she visits the house to collect and return the dog, she learns about dying; she does not need to talk about death in order to walk the dog (she just needs to like dogs), but walking the dog will teach her about death – just as offering to babysit will teach her about babies. She becomes, to use Ariès word, *familiar* with death, as almost all young humans have done until the twentieth century.

It seems unlikely that practical local action will emanate from metropolitan death cafés where urban strangers talk for an hour or two with other urban strangers and then go their separate ways. There are, however, other death café models. Dialog, a compassionate community initiative in the largely rural county of Dorset, offers death cafés in small market towns with the invitation 'Talk about death and grow our caring networks.' Here the aim is that talking together can lead to practical action. The Church of England has trialled a potentially similar model, **GraveTalk**, in some of its parishes; here people who already know each other within a local congregation discuss death, dying and funerals. To what extent GraveTalk has fostered practical end of life care initiatives within parishes has not, to my knowledge, been researched.

Porous institutions

Some of what critics condemn as death's medicalisation is, in fact, its institutionalisation. Kübler-Ross's (1969) seminal study – in which she talked to nearly 300 patients dying of cancer and which told the world about psychological and emotional processes that dying people often go through – was based in a large Chicago hospital. The 'stages of dying' she identified – denial, anger, bargaining, depression, acceptance – are precisely the emotions felt by new inmates as they enter any **total institution** and lose their previous identities (Goffman, 1961). So was she hearing about dying, or about becoming an institutional inmate? Or both? Both dying and hospitals, not to mention care homes, impose losses with which the person has to come to terms.

The total institution, as identified by sociologist Erving Goffman, is in its pure form total. But many residential institutions, such as boarding schools and eldercare homes, are less than total – to a greater or lesser degree, residents may, for example, retain their own clothes, hairstyles, and possessions; come and go; receive visitors. In other words, the boundary between institution and outside world can be somewhat porous. I have visited elderly friends and relatives in porous care homes and retirement villages where some residents are more part of the local community than are some housebound elderly living in their own home. Goffman (1961), Townsend (1964) and others long ago revealed the potentially de-humanising effects of *total* institutions. It is therefore worth asking not only how dying may become more a natural community/family event rather than a medical event, but also if and how the institutional settings in which dying people often find themselves could become more porous, that is, inclusive of the person's own social networks and the wider community. Some, though, will always need an 'asylum', a haven where they are protected from the outside world, not least from their own family.

Death and community

Sociologists and anthropologists from Durkheim (1915) onwards have shown how, though death disrupts or even shatters the groups to which humans belong – from families, to communities, to entire nations – the social response to death is paradoxically one of the main motors of human society. As Peter Berger (1969: 52) said, human society comprises people 'banded together in the face of death'. More specifically, I have witnessed time and again in my own street how neighbourly support for dying residents has brought neighbours together, creating bonds that then may last decades (Walter, 1999a). In other words, social capital and social networks are not a limited resource that, when called upon, necessarily get depleted. Rather, the opposite: using them can extend and strengthen them (Horsfall et al, 2011).

Affluence enables people to lead ever more independent lives. With every household owning a washing machine, fridge and freezer, more than one car and several digital communication devices, the need for launderettes, small local shops, buses and cinemas, along with the social encounters they foster, steadily declines. Yet bodies remain vulnerable, in need of hands-on attention: babies, pets and those nearing the end of life have physical needs that require a resident carer or carers, who at times need the extra support of those who live nearby, that is, neighbours. Using a neighbour to babysit, feed the cats for the weekend, or sit with your dying husband as you go to the pharmacy requires you to know your neighbours *and* helps you get to know them, to build up reciprocal obligations: 'Thanks for helping me out. Do let me know any time I can help you.' Sociologist Michael Young, one of the architects of the post-war British welfare state and doyen of community studies, toward the end of his long life interviewed people dying of cancer in London's East End. He concluded: 'Death is *the* common experience which can make all members of the human race feel their common bonds and their common humanity' (Young and Cullen, 1996, 201).

Questions

- **Discuss the four professional roles outlined in this chapter.**
- **What challenges need to be overcome for formal services at end of life to coordinate with bottom-up action within the local community?**
- **How could my city/neighbourhood/employer/church support healthy dying, caring and grieving?**

Notes

[1] www.who.int/healthpromotion/conferences/previous/ottawa/en/index4.html
[2] Chapter Eight describes how social media can contribute to reducing isolation among housebound elderly people.
[3] Thus the 2017 Dying Matters campaign not only urged Britons to talk about dying but also challenged them to consider 'What can you do?'.

FIVE

Why hold a funeral?

This chapter examines a contemporary trend in Anglophone societies toward seeing the funeral as a celebration of the deceased's unique life, rather than or as well as a religious rite or as a display of family status. This trend raises questions about the funeral industry's structure and about funeral poverty. Britain is taken as the case study.

Life-centred funerals

Sociologists, anthropologists, historians and archaeologists have highlighted two factors (among others) that shape funerals in any human society – religion and socio-economic status. How these have influenced funerals in Anglophone societies in recent centuries will now be explored, focusing on the contemporary shift toward a more secular society and toward greater economic security.

Religious change

Put simply, funerals in western societies that once looked forward, helping the deceased's soul on its way, increasingly look backward, celebrating the life that was lived on earth. This shift began in the seventeenth-century Protestant Reformation. By maintaining that

Christians get to heaven through their own faith and through God's grace, the Reformers made clear that neither the family's nor the church's prayers could assist the dead. At very most, the Protestant funeral could commend the deceased to God; seventeenth-century English and Scottish Puritan funerals were therefore very short and ritually 'thin', leaving something of a vacuum. In time this came to be filled in various ways such as expressing grief through melancholic poetry and the contemplation of nature (Draper, 1967) and, for those who could, demonstrating the deceased's social status through putting on a sumptuous post-funeral feast (Gittings, 1984). By the nineteenth century, intellectuals were challenging the existence of hell, and by the end of the twentieth century very few English-speaking people outside the USA and Ireland (North and South) believed in it (Walter, 1996). If heaven is the automatic destination, then funeral and mourning rites really have no spiritual work to do, even for Catholics.

By the late twentieth century, most Anglophone countries were becoming less religious, at least in a creedal sense, including by the twenty-first century even Ireland and to some extent the USA, though belief in heaven and a soul has remained buoyant. Religious funeral rites based on a seventeenth-century prayer book that made little or no mention of the life lived came to seem increasingly out of touch. So, late twentieth-century funerals began to become more personal, such that now many people expect the funeral to be a celebration of life – often called a personal or life-centred funeral (Garces-Foley and Holcomb, 2005). Increasing numbers of funerals in Australia, New Zealand and now the UK are led not by a minister of religion, but by a celebrant representing no religious organisation who works with the family to co-produce a unique celebration of the person's life (which may or may not include religious or spiritual elements). Funerals led by ministers of religion typically now include a eulogy or tribute to the deceased, spoken by either the minister or family or friends – these funerals look both forward and backward (Cook and Walter, 2005).

Economic change

Industrialisation entails agrarian populations migrating to rapidly expanding industrial cities to become paid factory and service workers. This involves not just geographical mobility, but moving into an entirely new kind of society, typically generating intense **status anxiety**, not to mention **economic insecurity**. In response, the funeral may become a display of family respectability, with spending on material accoutrements (coffin, hearse, horses/cars and so on) reflecting the family's means. Underlying this for poorer families in Victorian Britain was fear of a **pauper funeral** (Richardson, 1989). In the twentieth century, funeral expenditure driven by status insecurity may be seen in the 'baroque' American funerals critiqued for their extravagance by the uncomprehending upper-class British writer Jessica Mitford (1963); in the even more expensive funerals of rapidly modernising Japan (Bernstein, 2006); and in the rapidly expanding cities of West Africa (Jindra and Noret, 2011).

Unprecedented expansion of the British middle class in the mid-twentieth century meant that many people's social status became secure, no longer needing expression in the funeral. Most middle-class funerals became a lot simpler, as it subsequently turned out, perhaps too simple. From the late 1980s, moves to make bland British funerals more meaningful (Walter, 1990) have focused not on the family's material status but on the deceased's unique life and character. I call these 'postmaterial' funerals. **Postmaterialism** (Inglehart, 1981) refers to the personally expressive values of people who feel economically secure – very different from the values of people struggling to survive. The latter were of course dominant in the industrial revolution that gave birth to the British funeral industry and its material trappings of display. This helps explain why today many immigrant and working-class funerals are often more elaborate than middle-class ones. Some working-class funerals today display both status *and* personal character: lavish expenditure plus creative personalisation, a good send-off that is both material and personal.

Putting religious and economic change together, the funeral's purpose has evolved from looking forward to heaven and displaying the family's ongoing social status, to looking back to celebrate the deceased's unique life. Some funerals do both, combining personal celebration with religious hope and/or status display. With some variations (Walter, 2005), this transformation may be seen in Australia, New Zealand, Britain, Canada and the USA.

Archaic structures?

As the funeral's purpose has evolved, entrepreneurs offer new products and services. The funeral industry has adapted easily to some of these and not at all to others, as will now be discussed in the British context.

In pre-industrial Britain, the family would inform the vicar of the death, buy a coffin from the local carpenter, and borrow the village hand-bier. During the industrial revolution, many carpenters and hauliers added to their work the role of undertaker, now **funeral director** (FD), becoming the family's main contractor. He dealt directly with coffining, storing and transporting the body, and subcontracted out the religious service. With the funeral as a display of economic status, the key questions were how elaborate the coffin and hearse were to be, how many horses, and so on. By contrast, the religious service required little thought: Anglicans had the Anglican rite, Methodists the Methodist service, Catholics the Catholic mass, and within each rite, there was little or no choice apart from the hymns. So the major choices concerned material kit. The undertaker, who advised on this and sold much of it himself, was therefore the appropriate contractor, the person to whom the family went to arrange everything; he subcontracted out services he did not provide himself, such as the religious service and the burial plot. Victorian undertakers were heavily criticised, not least by novelist Charles Dickens, for trading on people's insecurities and promoting unnecessary expenditure; so in time, while still purveying material kit, they recast themselves as custodians of the body and overseer/controller of the whole funeral process, roles they continue to this day (Howarth, 1996).

For many of today's families, however, the major decisions are about how to personalise the ceremony. With this shift in focus from the body and its accoutrements to the ceremony, it would seem more logical for families first to consult a ceremony expert, who would then subcontract out the work of coffining, storing and transporting the body. Yet the industry's structure in which pole position of main contractor is occupied by a purveyor of material kit, namely the FD, remains intact; families therefore typically make key decisions with an FD who is more concerned with and more knowledgeable about hardware than ceremony. This structure, fit for Victorian status display, is arguably no longer fit for personalised ceremonies. However, not only do FDs not want to give up pole position, but also few ceremony workers (clergy, celebrants, and others) would wish to have ultimate responsibility for everything, including the body. Clergy in particular have parishes to run as well as the occasional funeral to conduct and are in no position to turn themselves into small businesses.

So, this leaves an industry structure intended for status display through material goods struggling to serve mourners who wish to focus on personal memories. This is reflected in the pricing of funerals. Of the average £3,700 cost for a 'basic funeral',[1] only £200 goes to the minister or celebrant, together with about £400 for hire of the ceremony venue (usually the crematorium chapel), printing of the ceremony programme and so on. The remaining £3,000 goes on material kit (coffins, vehicles, cremators), FD and crematorium overheads and care of the body.

Since the 1990s the demand for more personal funerals has driven significant new products and services. Some – such as natural burial grounds, companies providing personalised coffins, and freelance celebrants – have succeeded. That is because they accept their role as subcontractors to the FD, who thus has more services to offer the family, which in turn enhances his role as overall event manager.

Other innovations, however, have struggled because they challenge the FD's position as contractor-in-chief. Celebrants who have invited families to come first to them to devise the ceremony, subcontracting body care and transport to FDs, have unsurprisingly been blocked by FDs. The few who succeeded only did so because they turned themselves into FDs. More recently, however, some new start-up FDs competently arrange both ceremony and hardware with their clients, offering a seamless service. Some existing FDs now provide their own in-house celebrant, so could – in theory though not always in practice – provide a similarly integrated service.

Direct cremation

At the time of writing (2017), the most significant innovation in British funeral rites (or non-rites), imported from the USA, is direct cremation – the body is cremated with no prior viewing, no cortege and no funeral ceremony. It is relatively easy to set up a direct disposal business – all you need is an unmarked van and somewhere on an industrial estate to store bodies before you transport them to the crematorium. David Bowie's direct cremation in early 2016 cost $700. In the UK, costs range from £1,000 to £1,500.[2] With body disposal separated from ceremony, families are free – if they want – to hold a memorial service some days or weeks later.

Why choose direct cremation? Avoiding the pomp of a motor cortege and a full funeral service was the motive for direct cremation's original development in the USA several decades back and seems the most likely motive today in the UK – or at least in the absence of research, this is the picture emerging from anecdotal comments within the industry. Money is not usually the issue. Britons least able to pay the average £3,700 for a funeral are often those needing material display, that is, to arrange 'a good send-off', and who might feel ashamed of doing without the cortege and the funeral service. Direct cremation is therefore likely to appeal more to secure middle-class families who see no point in pomp and ceremony; certainly, this is the sales pitch of a number of direct cremation companies. It is the Bowies of this world who have manifestly gained respect and status in life who do not need to display it in death: just burn my body and go on enjoying my songs.

The flip side is that those who struggle to pay around £3,700 for a funeral are unlikely to go for the most radical way to reduce costs, namely to sidestep FDs with their fancy vehicles, coffins and corteges and to opt for direct cremation. This brings us to the contemporary issue of funeral poverty.

Funeral poverty

The British welfare state introduced a universal Death Grant in the late 1940s. Its original value was sufficient to pay for a simple funeral, but over the years failed to keep up with increases in funeral costs, and the grant was abolished in 1987. In its place, the Department for Work and Pensions' discretionary **Funeral Payment Scheme** now covers less than half the cost of a simple funeral, and the decision whether to award it is not made till many weeks after the funeral; it is therefore impossible for a hard-pressed family to make an informed decision as to what kind of funeral it can or cannot afford (Foster and Woodthorpe, 2013). At the time of writing, funeral poverty is increasing and has been highlighted by reform groups, the media and politicians (Work and Pensions Select Committee, 2016). Yet the most radical way to reduce funeral costs, namely sidestepping FDs and taking the body direct from place of death to place of disposal, does not feature in policy proposals to tackle funeral poverty. Why? The answer may be found on both supply and demand sides.

On the supply side, though the National Association of Funeral Directors urges its members to do their utmost to combat funeral poverty, it is unsurprising that they have not raised the possibility of families sidestepping them. On the demand side, those at risk of incurring funeral debt are by definition economically insecure and therefore more likely to want a funeral that displays their social respectability through material expenditure (McManus and Schafer, 2014). Thus the legacy of the nineteenth century is a system that creates funeral poverty: an industry that depends on the sale of hardware and bodycare, and a culture in which the shame of the pauper funeral, or at least the need to 'put on a good show', haunts materially insecure families or at least some members of some families. If the structure of Britain's contemporary funeral industry is inappropriate for families for whom ceremony is more important than body care and material display, it is also inappropriate for those who struggle to afford a funeral. How then may funeral poverty be tackled?

Do-it-yourself funerals, in which the family dispenses with FD, celebrant and/or cemetery, is the most radical way to reduce costs, but is unlikely to be chosen by more than a very few. More significant are the following: public health funerals, council funerals, compassionate communities and cultural diffusion.

Public health funerals

An option that very few families choose is to refuse to dispose of the body, in which case the local council has a statutory obligation to bury or cremate it and then attempt to recover the cost from the estate. If the estate has no money, the council has to pay for this 'public health funeral' – the modern term for a pauper funeral. Outwardly the funeral looks no different from a very simple standard funeral and might therefore not attract stigma, though still remains unacceptable to many families.

Council funerals

Some councils have contracted with a particular local FD to offer families a cut-price 'council funeral'. Those provided by Cardiff, Nottingham and Hounslow, for example, cost about £2,000, including the cremation fee though not the minister or celebrant's fee. This option, however, severely reduces choice, not least the choice of FD, and the total cost may still exceed what the Funeral Payment Scheme can cover.

Compassionate communities

An entirely different model is for the community to arrange and/ or pay for the funeral. For example, a family in difficult economic circumstances provides for the deceased a culturally appropriate send-off, possibly including considerable material display, and the community helps the family pay for it, either by individual donations or by fundraising through a community event such as a 'fun day' in honour of the deceased. My own town's poorest neighbourhood has witnessed several examples of this; other UK examples are sometimes reported in local news media; in sub-Saharan Africa this approach is common (Jindra and Noret, 2011). Internet crowdfunding enhance the possibilities. In Japan, attenders at *any* funeral or the preceding wake donate a sum of money, termed *koden*, to the family, who in turn later reciprocate by giving the attender a smaller, material gift; this both helps pay for the funeral, and strengthens reciprocal ties with a wide range of people at just the moment when a key human tie has been sundered.

A different model is offered in the Derbyshire town of Darley Dale by its Community Funeral Society; the CFS is staffed by volunteers who subcontract body handling to the one local FD who understands that support between death and the funeral can be a community responsibility.[3] The CFS has similarities to volunteer-staffed Jewish burial societies. These examples all fit the 'compassionate community' concept (see Chapter Four), in which the end of life is seen as a community responsibility, with the consequence that the grieving family gets integrated into the community rather than isolated from it.

Cultural diffusion

Perhaps the most effective long-term way to reduce funeral poverty is not through any specific policy or practice, but through the continuing cultural diffusion of the notion that a respectful funeral is one that commemorates or celebrates the deceased's unique life and personality. If this idea becomes more widely and deeply held, poorer families may come to question whether material display is necessary or expected. One blog about a DIY funeral admits how hard this can be:

> My grandmother grew up with the fear and shame poorer families felt about pauper burials... To be totally honest with

you, I did worry what people might think, and worried they would think we were doing the funeral on the cheap. I was shocked and horrified at how deep my conditioning went...I believe the kindness of all the official people involved helped us enormously to overcome our conditioning. Never once did we feel judged.[4]

If all those who attended this funeral also came away feeling positive, they too may come to question the necessity of material display. It is possible, but by no means inevitable,[5] that the idea that respect is better demonstrated through a life-centred ceremony than through material display could filter through to the poorest families. Funeral reformers before the late twentieth century attempted to cut material display without replacing it with anything, appealing only to the middle classes; might the life-centred ceremony now provide a meaningful replacement, even for the least well-off?

Question

How may funeral poverty best be tackled?

Notes

[1] www.sunlife.co.uk/press-office/cost-of-dying-2015/
[2] www.goodfuneralguide.co.uk/direct-disposal/
[3] http://communityfunerals.org.uk/the-darley-dale-cfs/
[4] Honouring Michael's Last Wishes: www.greenfieldcoffins.co.uk/about-us/latest-news/item/77-honouring-michael-s-last-wishes
[5] The 2015 Scottish Working Group on Funeral Poverty detected a 'developing belief' in 'a connection between the complexity and cost of a funeral and...respect and love for the deceased', http://data.parliament.uk/WrittenEvidence/CommitteeEvidence.svc/EvidenceDocument/Work%20and%20Pensions/Bereavement%20benefits/written/26543.html Section 4.1.2

SIX

How to dispose of bodies?

With global population growth and urbanisation, increasing numbers of living bodies exist in close proximity to one another; what happens to these bodies when they die? How are they to be disposed of? This question has challenged the authorities in pretty much every country experiencing rapid urbanisation. This chapter considers first some of the issues, before sketching some solutions that have been employed or are envisaged. Many of the issues have been framed in terms of hygiene, pollution and environmental protection. But as anthropologist Mary Douglas (1966) pointed out, such concerns cannot always be taken at face value; they often represent or symbolise something else. We therefore have to keep our wits about us as we explore this particular terrain.

Issues

Hygiene

As urban populations expanded in the late eighteenth and early nineteenth century, several European countries experienced a burial crisis. The medieval system of rural churchyard burial, in which old bones unearthed while digging new graves were re-buried or placed in an ossuary, failed as urban gravediggers found themselves unearthing decomposing flesh. With the miasma theory of disease pointing to graves as a source of sickness, reformers identified a public health scandal and proposed an alternative. Cultural historian Thomas Laquer (2015) argues that, at least in England, this was an orchestrated moral panic, not supported by the facts. Rotting organic matter from the living – the faeces and urine of humans and animals, especially horses – along with food scraps weighed 200 times more than human corpses, and in many churchyards there was no quantum leap in the number of bodies. So why the sudden obsession with smells and health? Why had the dead suddenly become dirty and dangerous? Laquer's answer is that churchyards belonging to the established Church of England failed to meet the needs of non-conformists and atheists, who then used public health to undermine the Anglican monopoly. French historian Ariès (1981, 409–556) points to new bonds of affection within the family as the motive for a more respectful place of repose for the dead. Whatever the cause, throughout Europe a new concept emerged – the **secular cemetery** where a religiously diverse population could be buried without risk to the sensibilities or health of the living.

Today, two centuries later, burial reformers remain concerned about public health, but focus less on hygiene than on pollution – from cremation rather than burial. Crematoria emissions include vaporised substances from the coffin (veneers, synthetic handles) and objects placed within the coffin (teddy bears, toys), along with mercury teeth fillings – estimates of the proportion of airborne mercury in the UK emanating from crematoria have varied from 5 per cent to 16 per cent (DEFRA, 2003). Environmental legislation in Europe, such as the UK's 1992 Environmental Protection Act, now requires the scrubbing of crematoria emissions to remove harmful products.

Religious diversity

Cities bring diverse people together, along with their diverse cultural traditions and religious requirements about disposing of the dead. Thus, not only did nineteenth-century non-conformists lobby for secular cemeteries, but twenty-first century Muslims require graves to be oriented toward Mecca, and Hindus expect to witness the coffin entering the cremator, in each case requiring re-design or at least modification of cemeteries and crematoria.

Respect

Though disposing of a body is a very physical matter, it is also – for those connected to the deceased – highly emotional, eliciting not only grief but also concerns about the fate of the soul. As anthropologist Robert Hertz (1907) argued over 100 years ago, subsequently confirmed in several studies of traditional societies, the fate of body, soul and mourners are closely and symbolically related. Human feelings of respect for the dead and respectful disposal of the body can be complex, related to formal religion, folk religion and personal psychology.

Filial respect has been central to Chinese culture for millennia. The most loving filial act is to bury your parents and worship them as ancestors, expressed in rituals at the grave at certain prescribed times of the year. In contemporary Chinese cities experiencing massive in-migration, the authorities are currently re-locating the contents of between 10 and 15 million graves at quite short notice, causing a degree of distress. Cremation became the only option in some cities in 2014, resulting in some elderly Chinese people committing suicide in order to get buried before the regulation was enacted, hence ensuring their post-mortem status as ancestors.[1]

Yet people are often able to adapt traditional notions of respect to new circumstances. In Singapore, where only one cemetery remains operational and cremation is encouraged, ancestral rites evolve in conjunction with new facilities, including ultra-modern visitor-friendly columbaria for storing ashes. In Britain, Hindus have adapted the traditional custom practiced in India of the eldest son breaking open the deceased's skull half way through the open pyre cremation; British Hindus insist simply on witnessing the coffin being slid into the modern gas cremator. Respect, rites, and disposal technologies all adapt to each other (Aveline-Dubach, 2012).

Ecology

Today in many western countries, ecological discourse dominates disposal of the dead. Here the concern, ostensibly, is not pollution directly affecting mourners or neighbours, but wider impacts on the planetary environment, including carbon emissions. In the USA, where burial of elaborate caskets in concrete-lined vaults has until very recently been the standard mode of disposal, one environmentally aware website advises potential funeral customers that 'About 800,000 gallons of formaldehyde-based embalming fluid are buried in US cemeteries every year. Ten acres of a typical cemetery contain nearly 1,000 tons of casket steel, 20,000 tons of concrete in burial vaults, and enough wood used in coffins to build 40 homes'.[2]

In the UK, it is crematoria that are under the spotlight, not least as their carbon emissions can be easily monitored, whereas the methane – a far more powerful contributor to global warming than carbon dioxide – emanating from graves is very difficult to measure. Natural burial is assumed to be more ecological, though this is not necessarily the case: a natural burial to which mourners drive many miles may have a higher carbon footprint than a local cremation. And open funeral pyres in India are many times more polluting than modern gas or electric cremators. In one Indian province, emissions from funeral pyres have been estimated to comprise 'about 23 percent of the total carbonaceous aerosol mass produced by the burning of fossil fuels in the region' (Friedman, 2014).

Sustainability: disposal techniques

Disposal practices deemed respectful, hygienic or ecological are not always sustainable, as will become apparent as we now turn to different techniques for disposing of bodies.

European grave re-use

As already noted, the practice of re-using graves within village churchyards sustained the burial of Europe's dead for over a millennium until the population exploded two centuries ago. In the nineteenth century, continental Europe replaced the medieval policy of re-use with a more rational policy of re-use. Thus today a family now leases the grave for a specified period – in my experience as little as eight years in a village in the outskirts of Antwerp, and 30 years in parts of Finland. After this period, the family has the option to pay to renew the lease, or to relinquish it so that the grave may be re-used by others. In this way, the burial ground continues to generate income, and every grave is leased by a family with a current interest so is likely to be looked after by the family. Neglected graves are therefore rare. The increase in cremation, however, means that old graves are no longer replaced by new ones; removing the lease-expired stones has left some cemeteries in, for example, Denmark and Switzerland looking forlornly empty.

The British cemetery

Britain, which in the nineteenth century included all of Ireland, responded very differently. Guided by the popular garden journalist John Claudius Loudon's 1843 handbook, new cemeteries comprising permanent graves were constructed on the outskirts of each town. The British were to rest in peace six foot down, never to be disturbed – not least by the grave robbers who had been finding a ready market for their gruesome wares in the booming anatomy schools (Richardson, 1989). Loudon foresaw that, within a generation or two in fast expanding cities, each cemetery would become full and be surrounded by new suburban development; but planted with fine specimen trees and adorned with architect-designed sepulchral monuments, they would continue as green oases, visited on Sundays by the urban populace for their aesthetic and moral betterment. The local municipality, recognising the value of this, would pay for the upkeep of full cemeteries. To cater for new burials, Loudon envisaged a new cemetery being constructed on the new urban periphery, and so on, indefinitely into the future.

A brilliant plan, incorporating a sustainability strategy! But its anticipation of urban populations wanting green space within their ever-growing cities was all too accurate – cities began building urban parks. Soon the masses preferred to take their children and their dogs and their cricket bats and balls to the local park, not to the gothic cemetery. This left urban cemeteries high and dry. After a few decades, with few remaining graves left to sell, many private cemeteries got into financial difficulties and were taken over by municipalities who found themselves with a large swathe of urban land needing upkeep but of little use and generating little or no income. The burial crisis had thus shifted from a crisis of hygiene to one of finance.

The American lawn cemetery

The British cemetery assumed families would look after the graves. But after a few years grief lessens; after five, ten or twenty years, the closest mourners with most interest in looking after the grave have themselves died; or the family may move from the area. With no free labour and no money coming into the cemetery, graves became dilapidated and dangerous.

The USA, like the UK, developed a policy of permanent graves. But with American families moving hundreds or thousands of miles inter-state, cemetery companies knew they could not rely on the family to tend graves. This led to two innovations. First, graves were sold with a sum added for 'perpetual care' which was invested and enabled the cemetery company to do all the maintenance. Second came the invention of the lawn cemetery and then the memorial park where graves are marked minimally, for example by a small metal plaque flush to the ground, and the whole area grassed over. Maintenance therefore simply entails a weekly mow by an industrial lawnmower, paid for by the perpetual care fund (Sloane, 1991). More recently, however, the relative anonymity of such cemeteries, like the mid-twentieth century

British crematorium funeral, has prompted a reaction demanding greater personalisation.

Cremation

The British cemetery, eschewing both the continental European and the American systems for ensuring ongoing income and maintenance, became financially unsustainable. Britain therefore became the first western country in which cremation became the norm – not because mid-twentieth century Britons particularly wanted it or believed in it, nor because Britain was particularly short of space (re-use could have solved that), but because municipalities who had inherited unsustainable Victorian cemeteries chose to restore their finances by building crematoria (Jupp, 2006). At that time, the 1940s to the 1960s, relatively few Britons belonged to religious minorities (Roman Catholic, Eastern Orthodox, Muslim) opposing cremation, so there was little to stand in the municipalities' way. To this day, the European countries with the lowest cremation rates, such as Spain and Italy, are not the least crowded but the most monolithically Catholic or, as with Greece and Romania, Orthodox.

The history of cremation in the USA is entirely different. Cremation was introduced in the USA as direct disposal without any ceremony around the casket, enabling economically secure Americans to reject the pomp, ceremony and showy caskets of the mid-twentieth century baroque funeral (see Chapter Five). With Americans equating cremation with no funeral accoutrements and no service, it is not surprising that American funeral directors did their utmost to resist it – until the early 1990s when a few enlightened FDs realised that it would be better to make a few hundred dollars on a cremation than no dollars at all (Kubasak, 1990). Since then, as more and more FDs accept cremation, more and more families opt for it (Prothero, 2000). If in the UK cremation developed in the twentieth century as 'full service' and only in the twenty-first century has direct cremation become available, in the USA it has been the other way around.

New concepts: dispersal techniques

All the above techniques attempt to dispose of the body, to get rid of it. In contemporary environmental discourse, however, disposal – of anything – is never final (Hetherington, 2004). Waste disposal does not exterminate matter, but re-locates and/or transforms it. Even if disposal succeeds in removing waste solids and liquids, it is only to re-locate them underground, disperse them into the ocean, or turn them into gasses that may cause greenhouse warming; each affects the ecosystem. Environmental discourse thus changes the understanding of disposal, for nothing is got rid of 'forever'.

This discourse is now found in the British burial and cremation industry (Rumble et al, 2014). Since the 1990s, all disposal innovations – natural burial, heat recycling from crematoria, and proposals to dissolve or freeze-dry human remains – have been promoted by means of environmental rhetoric. Each of these innovations recycles the remains of the dead, transforming them and then dispersing them into the everyday environment – a feature which promotional material often highlights as a selling point.

Natural burial

Since 1993, well over 200 natural burial grounds (NBGs) have been established around the UK; these bury whole bodies and ashes in ground that is, or is intended to become, woodland or meadow. When full, the meadow or wood will become a part of the natural landscape; some NBGs will eventually become nature reserves managed by a wildlife charity or trust. The aim is to create a space that looks not like a burial space but one that looks, or will in time look, like a meadow or woodland full of local flora and fauna. In British natural burial discourse, human remains nourish nature and become part of the natural world that sustains the living (West, 2008; Davies and Rumble, 2012).

The word 'natural' should be understood symbolically rather than literally. The only natural place for large mammals to die and decompose is on the ground, there to be eaten by bugs, flies and scavengers. Burial under the ground is not natural but cultural. For many mourners, however, natural burial symbolises their or the deceased's values, or provides a setting which they feel comfortable visiting.

Several other English-speaking countries have their own versions of natural burial; in each country, the symbolism reflects specific national myths about nature. Raudon (2011, 18) argues that green burial in New Zealand is less about ecology than about getting close to nature – the bush, the outdoors: 'Perhaps in England it is considered one of the minor duties of good citizenship to give back to the world at the end of life while in New Zealand it is regarded as one of the rights of all citizens to lay claim to the land, even after death.' Similar meanings may apply in the USA, another immigrant society with a national mythology of white pioneers, empty land and fecund soil.

Cremation

Advocates of natural burial often portray it as the opposite of the modern cremator – a computer-controlled, high-tech furnace consuming large amounts of energy. Yet here too, environmentalism is driving new language, new technology and new operating practices. In response to financial inducements and legal requirements to protect the environment, the British cremation industry now cools emissions so that any mercury can liquefy and be removed; a few crematoria have used the heat available from this process – heat generated in large part by the burning body – to heat the crematorium chapel or nearby buildings. In addition, medical implants such as titanium hips are removed from the ashes and recycled. Thus cremation, like other forms of waste disposal, is no longer a simple matter of disposal but becomes instead a carefully managed process of re-use, while the burning body itself becomes useful for warming the living.

Alkaline-hydrolysis

Alkaline-hydrolysis – operational in several US states and actively promoted in the UK – was originally developed in the 1990s to dispose of animal carcasses. The process dissolves the dead body's organic matter in a stainless-steel container filled with water and potassium hydroxide; heat and pressure are added, reducing the body to a liquid that can then be recycled at the local waste-water treatment plan. Other proposed uses of the fluid include agricultural fertiliser. The small pieces of bone fragment that remain are crushed into 'ashes' and given to families, as in cremation; any remaining inorganic matter, such as mercury fillings or medical devices, can be recycled.

If alkaline-hydrolysis becomes a more widespread way to dispose of human bodies, we may find ourselves drinking water recycled from this process or eating food grown using fertiliser from human remains. It is hard to predict whether this will prove to be culturally acceptable, though market research in England and Scotland commissioned by Co-operative Funeralcare provides optimism (Thomas, 2010; 2011). The American state of New Hampshire changed its law to allow alkaline-hydrolysis, but then revoked this a few years later over concerns that human remains were being sent down municipal drains. A local newspaper provides a flavour of the arguments for and against:

> Supporters…did not object to the liquid residue being spread as fertilizer or flushed into the sewer. 'I would like to think someday I would give something back to this earth that gave me the life I have,' said Nottingham Republican Frank Case. Opponents said the process was disrespectful. 'I don't want to send a loved one to be used as fertilizer or sent down the drain to a sewer treatment plant,' said Bedford Republican John Cebrowski. (Love, 2009)

Freeze-drying (Promession/Cryomation)

Promession, invented by the Swedish ecological educator Susanne Wiigh-Mäsak and trademarked as Cryomation, uses liquid nitrogen to super-cool the body so it becomes friable and can be shaken into a kind of compost which, when shallow buried in soil, quickly converts into mulch. Its environmental credentials are highlighted: 'Cryomation will deliver a safer, more environmentally friendly option for people that sustains the life of the environment.'[3] The Promessa website is headed 'Promession – ecological burial', and depicts young shoots growing out of compost.[4] In countries such as the UK where human remains may legally be buried almost anywhere, a family could thus use a deceased member's remains as compost in their garden. Even in countries where the law would require the compost to be used in a legally designated burial ground, the image is still of humans becoming part of the natural cycle, symbolised not by a stone marking the dead but by new shoots creating new life for the living. There is as yet no country where this process is operational.

Private ash rituals

Another, more informal, change in British cremation practice prepared the rhetorical ground for the concept of dispersal. The private scattering and burial of ashes, legal in the UK though not in all countries, has become popular in recent decades (Prendergast et al, 2006; Hockey et al, 2007). Many families scatter or bury ashes in places that have personal meaning because of an association with life rather than with death: the back garden, a football ground, a favourite beach or mountain top. The ashes become part of an already cherished environment. But they are still deposited, *disposed* of, in these places.

The concept of dispersal is found, however, in other ash practices (Prendergast et al, 2006). One is when ashes are dispersed between various mourners, though arguably this is not so much dispersal as disposal in separate locations. More significant is the practice, engaged in not only by Hindus, of sprinkling ashes onto rivers or the sea, with the imagery of being dispersed into the planet's oceans. Finally, while the reality of scattering on land causes the ash to fall promptly to the nearby ground, the *image* of scattering 'to the winds' to become 'Part of all you see/The air you are breathing', to quote Ewan McColl's

1980s song *The Joy of Living* (performed at his cremation), clearly invokes a vision of dispersal.

Policy and law

Since the mid-nineteenth century, policies for disposing of the dead have been premised on their physical removal to cemetery or crematorium away from spaces occupied by the living. This is now being challenged, or at least supplemented, by the new concept of dispersal of remains into natural and/or everyday environments. So far, the British planning process and the courts have not opposed these new ways of processing the dead. German law, by contrast, requires whole bodies to be buried in a conventional grave within a designated churchyard or cemetery, so natural burial can only be for ashes and it may be that other innovations will not be easily accommodated legally and institutionally. In the USA, relevant laws are made state by state. Thus legal histories and frameworks make innovation more or less possible, depending on the jurisdiction.

Though proponents of these new technologies emphasise their benign effects on the physical environment, the major effect may prove to be on social attitudes. These technologies' contribution to reducing global pollution is easily outweighed by India's open pyres (Friedman, 2014) and their contribution to reducing greenhouse gasses is outweighed several thousand-fold by China's new coal-fired power stations, but they may well prompt western publics to think differently about not only the environment but also death. Indeed, it may be that these dispersal techniques are ultimately more about re-creating the boundary between the living and the dead than about the environment (Douglas, 1966; Howarth, 2000). The final chapter explores this possibility further.

Questions

Is ecological dispersal of bodies significant for the planet, or is it more a symbolic gesture by the funeral industry and/or by some mourners? What would you want for your own or a loved one's body, and why?

Notes

[1] http://library.stanford.edu/projects/chinesegraves
[2] www.sevenponds.com/after-death/environmental-impact-of-death
[3] www.cryomation.co.uk/whatIsCryomation.html [accessed 23 September 2016]
[4] www.promessa.se/?lang=en

SEVEN

How to mourn?

That humans grieve the deaths of those to whom they are attached seems pretty much universal. Two major cross-cultural reviews of a large number of anthropological studies found crying a response to bereavement in almost all societies (Rosenblatt et al, 1976; Eisenbruch, 1984). Yet being incapacitated by grief for an extended period of time is not compatible with survival of the species – mourners would soon get eaten by lions and their children starve. Genetic or cultural evolution would surely have selected against it. So why is grief such a common human experience? The academic consensus is that attachment between humans, especially those to whom one is genetically related, is vital not only for survival but also for group cooperation and culture, and grief is a by-product of personal attachment. Yet grief has to be moderated by the need to survive, and it seems that in many societies throughout history and pre-history people mourned in the first instance and then had to get on with life. This chapter focuses on how this tension between grieving and surviving, between emotions and economics, changes as societies become more affluent and economically secure, and how this leads to new norms about how to grieve.

Stroebe and Schut's **dual process model** of coping with bereavement (1999) illuminates this tension. They argue that mourners are confronted by two kinds of stress, each calling for a response: there is the pain of loss, and there is the need to rebuild life and adapt to a changed world. Mourners typically oscillate between the two, between being oriented to loss and to restoration, often finding it impossible to do both at once. There may be times, whether in the life of an individual, a family or an entire society, when restoration and survival have to take priority, and other times when loss can more readily be addressed. A society's culture may privilege one of these over the other, valuing stoicism and a stiff upper lip over the expression of emotion (Scheper-Hughes, 1992; Jalland, 2010), or defining mourning as an emotional, psychological process of confronting loss which has to be addressed – as is increasingly asserted in affluent western societies (Wortman and Silver, 1989).

In what follows, 'bereavement' or 'loss' refers to the state of having lost someone or something, 'grief' refers to what is felt, and 'mourning' refers to what is done (Lofland, 1985). Some Anglophone writers reserve 'mourning' for culturally required bereavement behaviour, but this could be taken to imply that grief's emotions are not influenced by culture, which is incorrect (Walter, 1999b). I generally use 'mourner' in preference to the less elegant terms 'bereaved person' or 'griever'.

For some decades, contemporary western norms about how to respond to bereavement have been, and still are, contested (Doka and Martin, 2002; Walter, 1999b). The specific questions this chapter addresses are: Should bereavement care focus on loss or restoration, on emotions or economics? Should grief be contained or expressed? Should we let go of the dead or live with them? Can individuals ever be free to grieve their own way? I pose these questions as 'either/or' and indeed both experts and general culture have sometimes seen them as opposed, but the most helpful answers may well be 'both'.

Emotions or economics?

Demographic, social and cultural changes suggest that grief is likely to be felt particularly intensely in modern western societies. First, general affluence and a welfare state mean that one major historical reason for not addressing personal loss, namely pre-occupation with physical survival, is much reduced. Second, personal exploration of grief is encouraged by the romantic construction of love as the meaning of life together with a cultural focus on the inner life that began with the invention of the novel in the eighteenth century and continues through to contemporary culture's concern with vulnerability (Furedi, 2004). Third, the nuclear family concentrates threads of connectedness in a few intimate relationships, which (because of unprecedented life expectancy) may last many decades, so attachments (with all their complexities) can be very strong. Siblings may share time on the planet for eight or nine decades, spouses for five or six decades, and children can be in their 50s or 60s when their parents eventually die (Lofland, 1985). For all these reasons, twentieth-century bereavement came to be constructed as the intensely personal, private emotional experience of losing an intimate – even if opinions differed as to if and how grief should be expressed.

As well as prompting emotional reactions, however, bereavement can lead to a change in identity (for example, from wife to widow), economic problems (loss of a breadwinner), social problems (loss of the spouse's friends), loss of power (death of a high-status husband), increase of power (the child is now the head of the family), or spiritual anguish and/or religious support. In unpublished teaching material, Susan LePoidevin therefore identified multiple dimensions of loss:

1. *Identity* How has the loss changed the person's concept of themselves, their values, self-esteem?
2. *Emotional* How does the person express their emotions, and how has their emotional equilibrium been affected?
3. *Spiritual* What meaning has the person ascribed to their loss? How has it affected the meaning of life? Have religious beliefs been a comfort, or discarded (inducing a further loss)?
4. *Practical* How is the person dealing with everyday tasks? What new tasks have to be learned?
5. *Physical* How is the person's health affected? [Are there] sleep, weight, stress-related symptoms?

6. *Lifestyle* Will the person have to move house, start work, lose their social life?
7. *Family/community* How will roles, inside and outside the family, change? What support is there in the community?

Le Poidevin argued that different dimensions may predominate in different individuals or at different times in their bereavement; the practitioner's task is to identify what is causing the person difficulties at the present time and to help them with this. Developed in the 1980s, her dimensions do not explicitly include the economic, but several of them clearly include restoration as well as loss.

Since the mid-twentieth century, bereavement practitioners and researchers, at least in the UK, have shifted focus from the economic dimension to the emotional and then more recently, to some extent, back to the economic. In the 1950s, married women's participation in the labour force in the UK (and in many other countries) was much lower than it came to be in later decades (Walsh and Wrigley, 2001); Peter Marris' (1958) study of London widows whose working-age husband had died found economic hardship to be a major concern. When Cruse Bereavement Care – the UK's internationally respected and leading bereavement charity – was founded in 1959 it saw widows' problems as mainly social and economic (Torrie, 1987). Its first Fact Sheets dealt with income tax, housing, health and diet, pensions, insurance, children's education and training for work. Only later did Cruse focus on psychological counselling; increased female participation in the labour force, expanded welfare benefits and a reduction in the death rate of working-age husbands had softened widowhood's economic impact. Also, Cruse evolved to encompass all kinds of bereavement, not least middle-aged women's loss of an elderly parent; these parentally bereaved adults might actually gain financially by the death yet find the personal loss very hard.

In the twenty-first century, bereavement organisations and research in the UK are once again paying attention to bereavement's economic aspects (Corden and Hirst, 2013), possibly reflecting the erosion of welfare benefits to assist with bereavement and with funeral costs

(Foster and Woodthorpe, 2013), but also the practicalities of managing alone. Stroebe and Schut's (1999) dual process model of grief, picturing an oscillation between emotional pain and the socio-economic challenge of rebuilding life, has been well received by researchers and therapists, supplementing Freudian and attachment models which focus on emotional processes (Bowlby, 1961). In a recent study of the experiences of Britons whose partner had recently died, 22 per cent said that the financial impact of lower income was the most difficult aspect, with considerably more women affected than men; 16 per cent found it challenging to look after the house; 34 per cent found it difficult to cook; 37 per cent struggled with the washing and ironing (Trajectory, 2016). This may reflect a gendered division of labour. Older mourners are under-represented in this particular sample, but it seems likely that as ageing or disabled bodies prompt re-division of household labour, practical vulnerabilities in bereavement will increase further (Pincus, 1976). An older couple may manage because his non-arthritic wrists can open tins and bottles while her higher energy levels enable her to cook, but the death of one – especially the fitter one – leaves the other struggling. Such are the practical challenges faced by elderly widows and widowers living on their own in contemporary Britain, a country where – unlike the USA or Australia – removal to communal living is generally made only as a last resort.

Some consequences of the relation between economic and personal loss are explored in the next section.

Contain or express grief?

In time of war, even relatively affluent societies may expect stoicism. In the trenches of the First World War, soldiers could not fall apart in grief when their best mate was blown to bits; instead, they sang:

'Pack up your troubles in your old kit bag
and smile, smile, smile'

This was also expected of bereft mothers, wives and fiancées back home; they had to continue to work in the munitions factories or on the land to keep the war effort going. There was little space for grief. Historian Pat Jalland (2010) has argued that in the Second World War the famous Blitz spirit was not, or not just, a natural response to the need to keep fighting. It was carefully orchestrated by Prime Minister Winston Churchill who ensured that newspaper pictures and cinema newsreels depicted the sturdy air raid warden pulling an old woman out of the rubble and handing her a cup of tea, or the milkman continuing on his rounds through destroyed streets – very different from today's news coverage of bombing and disaster which highlights gaunt, dazed and distraught victims who are asked by interviewers how they feel about having lost home and family. Churchill intended both to convince the British that they could take whatever the Luftwaffe threw at them, and to convince Hitler – who would see these media images – that he could not bomb the Brits into submission. As propaganda, manipulating grief, it was brilliant. And it continued to influence the British for another generation.

After the Second World War, every badly bombed country had to re-build, focusing on restoration rather than loss (Stroebe and Schut, 1999). In Germany, there was no call to dwell on loss, whether of family members, of the Nazi ideals that millions had embraced, or the multitude of lives those ideals had destroyed (Mitscherlich and Mitscherlich,1975); not until the 1990s were the complexity of such issues publicly addressed.

More generally, however, the 1960s saw the stirrings of a reaction against stoicism, especially in English-speaking countries. Young baby boomers came to consider it healthy to express emotions of hurt and pain; repression, despite the psychological functions that Freud had shown it could play, came to be seen as unhealthy. This revised view was carried particularly by women working in what Bernice Martin (1981) has called the **expressive professions** (such as social work, healthcare, counselling), taking longer to influence men, the working class and the commercial middle class. Currently, opinion about the best way to handle stress, hurt and pain, including grief, is split –

between Churchillian stoics (often older, often male) and baby-boomer expressivists (Walter, 1999b).

Though there is some evidence that some men may benefit by being helped to express their emotions (Schut et al, 1997), evidence that expressing grief is good for mental health, as measured by standard psychological tools, is not as overwhelmingly positive as many in the expressive professions like to think; in fact, much of the evidence is mixed and inconclusive (Bonanno, 2004) and this has been known for at least 30 years (Wortman and Silver, 1989). This does not mean that bereaved people should not openly express their grief, nor that they should contain their feelings. People have the right to feel and do as they wish, without every emotion and behaviour being assessed in terms of psychological health. Grief is a natural human reaction, not a mental illness. Mental health should not be allowed to define good grief, any more than medical expertise should define a good death.

This does, however, present a challenge for those who work in healthcare. Since they are employed to care for people's health, they should think hard before promoting interventions that have not been demonstrated to improve, or at least not harm, physical and mental health. An instructive case was the furore that followed Hughes et al's (2002) carefully designed study assessing hospital guidelines that mothers whose child is stillborn benefit from seeing and holding the dead child. The researchers found that a year later mothers who had seen their child were more anxious and had more symptoms of trauma than those who had not seen their child, while those who had in addition held their stillborn were more depressed. The researchers carefully outlined the study's limits, but pointed out that – in the absence of any other studies to date – the guidelines should be reassessed (which eventually happened in the UK). For the time being, mothers who wanted to see and hold their dead child could of course do so, but they should not be encouraged, and certainly not be told it would help them. The hostile reaction to this cautiously worded report suggests that the guidelines had been based on personal experience, anecdotal evidence, and passionate belief which its advocates were loath to give up. Evidence-based medicine, however, requires those who work in healthcare to advocate practices that demonstrably improve mental or physical health (Halpern, 2015).

Two views on the value of expressing grief may be identified. One is that the cultural shift from stoicism to expressivism represents progress and that stoics who 'bottle up' their grief will sooner or later pay psychological consequences. This, for example, is the view of the historian Pat Jalland. An alternative view, which I hold, is that stoicism is an appropriate response in times of economic hardship and war, while expressing grief is more appropriate in economically and politically secure societies – though there will of course be differences from person to person. But if an affluent community experiences a disaster, a stoicism born of the need to survive may reappear for as long as everyone in the community has to work together to restore the basic services needed for survival. We now know that psychological counselling, of considerable value to the minority who continue to struggle personally once the immediate shock has passed and basic services have been restored, has little or no value in the immediate aftermath of disaster or indeed of any death (Bonanno, 2004; Schut and Stroebe, 2005; Currier et al, 2008).

Let go of the dead, or live with them?

The answer to this question has been shaped by two contradictory strands within western culture over the past two centuries (Stroebe et al, 1992; Walter, 1999b). The romantic movement celebrated love for spouse and children; love could not perish, it was eternal, lasting beyond the grave. Starting with romantic novels and poetry, this motif continued through grand opera and into twentieth-century pop songs, and is found over many decades in newspaper death notices, death anniversary notices and on gravestones. As a beautifully carved 1960 stone for an 11-year-old boy in an English country churchyard states:

'Brief is life but love is long'

And another stone, in Kensal Green Cemetery, London (1998):

'Those you love don't go away
They walk beside you every day'

This idea is also expressed in the twentieth century's most popular afterlife belief – soul reunion (Walter, 1996). This sees humans as comprising body and soul; the body will die, at which point the immortal soul proceeds to heaven where it is united with pre-deceased loved ones. Heaven thus consists of related souls enjoying each other's company, rather than unrelated souls worshipping their Maker (McDannell and Lang, 2001). Back on earth, when the second spouse's name is added to the gravestone, the inscription 'Together at last' is often added.

In tension with this romantic understanding is the 'modernist' understanding of the psychiatrists and psychologists who became the twentieth century's experts in bereavement. From Freud (1917) through Bowlby (1961) to Worden (1983), the message has been that the mourner has a goal: to detach from the painful emotions of loss so that she can once again become an autonomous individual, free to contract new relationships with other autonomous individuals. Through sexual union, birth and parenting, humans become attached to one another, and grief is the pain of those attachments being sundered; in modernist grief psychology, the pain has to be worked through so that the mourner can become reconstituted as a free individual. Mourners are to 'let go', 'move on'; the goal is 'closure'; grief is to be 'resolved'. The dead, like the old and the past, are to be left behind. Modernist grief psychology is of course more subtle than this, but given a twentieth-century culture that emphasised progress and the future, the message that entered popular culture was 'let go' and 'move on'.

Capitalism requires both a consumer ethic in which consumption enhances family love and happiness (Campbell, 1987), and a producer ethic valuing hard work (Weber, 1930); the first creates a demand for ever more goods, the second helps produce the goods. At home people are expected to be expressive, loving and committed for life; at work they are expected to be instrumental, to seek advancement up the career ladder and/or be flexible to seek employment elsewhere. The consumer ethic of loving, consuming families underlies the romantic understanding of bereavement, while the producer ethic that bans sentimentality and irrationality underlies the modernist imperative to let grief go and move on. It is hardly surprising that a capitalist economy that requires both ethics should generate a grief culture comprising two ethics; but whereas the two capitalist ethics complement each other and enable capitalism to function, the two bereavement ethics contradict each other and complicate grief.

Twentieth-century mourners thus found themselves caught between romantic and modernist expectations. But as the twentieth century drew to a close, there arose in some (not all) mature industrial societies a general re-valuing of roots, of heritage, of old buildings, of the past. Householders began to restore old furniture and old properties, town planners who had once condemned Victorian housing as slums came to re-define it as heritage, postmodern architects re-worked traditional motifs; all wanted to march into the future, not turning their back on the past but in its company. The past married to the future came to be seen both as profitable and as socially, ecologically and psychologically healthy. In this new context, experts changed their advice on whether to march into the future with, or without, the dead. In bereavement research, this has been expressed since the mid-1990s in the concept of '**continuing bonds**' in which mourners often retain a relationship to the dead – they can move on *with* the dead (Klass et al, 1996). Of course, many mourners already knew this, but the experts have perhaps now caught up. Thus, expert theories as much as popular assumptions are influenced by culture.

Freedom to grieve?

Many societies have strong norms as to how people should grieve, while most religions prescribe rituals to be conducted for the soul on specified days during the weeks, months and years following a death. Protestant Christianity, for reasons discussed in Chapter Five, is rather unusual in offering few if any such rites. And many contemporary western societies, as Chapter Three discussed in the context of dying, celebrate individual freedom and personal autonomy. Many westerners therefore feel grief should reflect not community or religious expectations but the griever's unique personal attachment to the deceased. Bereaved people should be free to grieve in whatever way feels right and natural to them. This is supported by attachment theory (Bowlby, 1981; Parkes, 2008) which argues that how a person grieves a particular death depends on the attachment styles s/he developed from infancy, together with the specific relationship s/he had with the deceased.

Why then might an economically secure society promoting freedom of expression discourage overt expression of grief, at least in certain settings? Doka and Martin (2002) contrast different personal grieving styles – instrumental and /intuitive – which to some extent resemble Stroebe and Schut's restoration and loss orientations, and this chapter's stoicism and expressivism. Reynolds (2002) suggests that modern work organisations, privileging instrumental ways of working, may disallow expressive/intuitive grieving styles in the workplace. We might theorise this using Foucault's concept of 'disciplinary power' (Foote and Frank, 1999) or Holst-Warhaft's (2000) argument that throughout history powerful institutions have suppressed grief in order to dampen its disruptive potential.

Another set of norms specifies not how to grieve, but who to grieve. Thus, the death of spouse, child or parent is expected to elicit more grief than that of a nephew, friend, colleague or animal companion. Such 'hierarchies of grief' have been challenged as 'disenfranchising' certain kinds of loss (Doka, 1989). The word 'disenfranchise', implying loss of citizenship, is significant: 'disenfranchised grief' is a concept employed in free democracies which believe in personal liberty. And indeed, in England, some of the late-Victorian women who challenged norms requiring ladies to grieve certain deaths (for example, their father-in-law's) longer than others (for example, their own baby's), were the same women who supported the suffragette movement (Taylor, 1983).

Can such hierarchies be so easily dispensed with, however? Robson and Walter (2012–13) showed how hierarchies of loss are understood and approved of, even by people who acknowledge grief to be unique and personal. And it seems unlikely that employers will abandon compassionate leave policies which allow more time off for the death of a spouse or a child than for the death of a distant cousin or companion animal (Kamerman, 2002). Those who argue that all grief should be enfranchised seem to be arguing for a society without norms; no such society has yet existed.

To conclude, compared to those who have lived in other societies, contemporary westerners have considerable freedom to grieve who and how they want. At the same time – precisely because of their love of freedom – they may resent what norms remain. This may be contrasted with most past societies where mourners understood and accepted that grief is subject to social norms, and that the policing of grief reflects society's structures of power.

Question

What principles should guide bereavement policy – for a workplace, a school, or a benefits system?

EIGHT

Distance and the digital:
how to connect?

The past decade has seen an explosion of research papers about social media mourning (Brubaker et al, 2013). Instead of simply summarising their findings, this chapter focuses on a specific tension in dying and grieving in a digital age: death is highly material, with the dying person, the funeral and the grave all sited in a particular geographical location, yet families may be geographically dispersed across a country or indeed the globe. Migration and geographic mobility, whether to live, to work, to retire, for asylum, or a gap year, put a physical distance between some family members and the dying person, the grave, and other family members – a distance that can be acutely felt. At the same time, digital social media keep migrants in touch with an immediacy inconceivable two centuries ago when sailing ships took many months to deliver a message from one end of the globe to the other. In death as in life, more humans today move great physical distances than ever before yet can be instantly in touch. How, then, do digital social media change the end of life, caring, dying, funerals and mourning? This chapter concerns death, distance and the digital – how physical distance and virtual presence interact at end of life. This includes how digital media can now also reduce social distance (of mourners from each other) and spiritual distance (of the dead from the living).

Distance

Distance has long been a factor in the experience of both birth and death. The city of ancient Rome at its peak had a population of around one million; many of its inhabitants had family members spread across the Empire. Indeed, most empires have entailed the mass movement of people, often including the deportation of thousands of slaves to new lands. The expansion of European power from the sixteenth century depended on colonists, merchants, sailors and slaves traversing the oceans in vessels that took months to cover distances that today are completed in hours by plane, and instantly by Skype. An exchange of letters between colonist and home could take a year of more, so the death of a close family member was heard about months afterwards, and attending the funeral out of the question. Slaves never heard from home.

The American Civil War (1861–65) saw two technology-driven innovations affecting death and mobility. First, the telegraph enabled news of death on the battlefield to reach the family in just hours. Second, railroads spurred the development of embalming techniques that could preserve bodies long enough for the rail journey home to a family funeral. Since then, further advances in both travel and communication now enable news to be imparted instantly and enable the living to visit the dying and the dead.

How death and dying interact with distance depends considerably on geography, resources and legal status. In countries such as England, the 'double burden' of caring for both teenage children and ageing parents prompts thousands of the already-busy middle-aged to drive each weekend from one end of the country to the other on congested motorways to check up on frail elderly parents and to organise and re-organise care packages that seem as fragile as their client. North Americans may consider driving many hours to visit family as normal; others may fly; or stay at home and Skype (Moore, 2012). In the

Netherlands, where almost everywhere is within two hours' drive or train journey, the double burden is objectively less. But how people *feel* about fitting all this travelling into already busy lives depends on subjective perception of distance: a Dutch person may find an hour's drive more stressful than an American's four-hour drive.[1]

For families whose members migrate intercontinentally, modern travel and modern communications present new choices and new dilemmas. If I book an expensive and exhausting flight from my home in New Zealand to visit my dying father in Scotland, will I get there in time? Can I afford a last-minute flight from Costa Rica to New York? If not, who in the family can I ask to help pay? Do we delay the funeral to enable relatives to book flights from the other side of the world – or do we link them to the funeral via webcasting or Skype? Do we take the ashes home? In any case, where is home – in Toronto where the deceased's children are, or Surinam where his parents and ancestors are (van der Pijl, 2016)?

As in past centuries for sailors, merchants, colonists and slaves, some migrants do not have the luxury of such choices. Vanessa Bravo (2017) describes the position of undocumented migrants in the USA whose mother or father lies dying in Latin America; if they return home to visit, they may not be able to get back into the USA where reside both their children and the job that enables them to support the extended family in Latin America. Those granted political asylum in the USA experience comparable uncertainties, for if they return to their home country, they risk arrest. For these migrants, Facebook, WhatsApp and especially Skype provide the only way to visit their dying relative – virtually. This is better than nothing, but does not erase the pain of being unable to go home.

Living in two worlds

Maurice Bloch's (1971) study of death rites in Madagascar showed how Malagasy people live in two worlds – the everyday world of global capitalism in which they physically live, and the symbolic world of the ancestors represented by the family's ancestral tomb-house. We may extend this notion beyond Bloch's original context, for migrants also typically live in two worlds – the place to which they have moved which provides practical economic and educational opportunities, and the place from which they have moved which symbolises family and roots.

When I visited Kenya in 1992, I found the roads out of Nairobi congested every Friday evening as thousands of the city's residents travelled for the weekend back to the *shamba*, the family farm where reside the old folk and the dead. Though many now get buried in Nairobi, the ideal in some ethnic groups is to be buried back home; the packed buses driving out of town convey the dead as well as the living. My distinct impression of Nairobi was not of a city of three million inhabitants but of millions of campers whose true home is somewhere else; living and working in the city, their hearts are elsewhere.

Serbian economic emigrants expect to return home, so do not plan to die in, for example, France or the USA, but may well do so. As the funeral oration for an American Serb eloquently stated, his soul 'goes to the Serbian heaven, while his body lies in this hospitable American land' (Pavicevic, 2009, 239). Even in more settled England, people can live in two, all-too physical, worlds – the everyday world of job, mortgage, friends and troubled teenage children in Southampton, and another world of incontinence pads, inadequate care packages and signs of dementia in the parental home six hours north in Lancashire.

I now sketch how living in two worlds operates at end of life, and the role of digital and social media. I consider dying, the remains, inheritance, mourning, and relationships with the dead.

Dying

Being there, or 'presence' (Chapter Four), is one of the roles that family members can play at the dying person's bedside, and visual social media such as Skype considerably enhance possibilities for presence compared to older communication technologies such as email, telephone or letter (Moore, 2012). As a supplement in between actual physical visits, virtual presence can be highly valued. As a substitute when physical visits are not possible, as with the undocumented migrants Bravo interviewed, it can be bittersweet, reminding both parties of physical separation and the absence of physical touch.

If social media can provide social and emotional support, they cannot provide hands-on care. However globalised my living, my dying needs people near enough to care for my body, to cook, to walk the dog. With family members dispersed around the country or around the globe, with professional care services stretched, and dying trajectories getting ever longer, the need for compassionate local communities is likely to increase, as discussed in Chapter Four.

Dispersed family and friends, however, are increasingly using social and digital media to coordinate care; software for organising diaries and schedules is available for families and carers. A son who lives many hours away thus goes online and finds that a neighbour will be calling to check on his mother at 10 am, while a good friend will be visiting in the afternoon; so the son schedules his phone or Skype call for the early evening.

It is much more challenging, however, to use this kind of software to coordinate care by family and friends with care by formal agencies. Health and social care agencies cite confidentiality to justify not giving outsiders access to their electronic systems; and they rarely encourage staff to participate in family-organised social media. I know of only one example where this has, to an extent, succeeded. A widow in her eighties with dementia, living at home with a live-in carer, has an adult son two hours away and a daughter five hours away. The daughter persuaded her mother's carer to use a shared online calendar for appointments such as shopping, going to the dentist and social visits so that friends and neighbours know when and when not to visit. In addition, son, daughter and (less often) the carer occasionally write in a shared online journal to record behavioural changes as the dementia develops, along with notes, pictures and music of happy times such as singing together or a birthday party, which overseas relatives appreciate. Using 'soft' surveillance, these shared online platforms improve quality of life for all concerned.

Digital surveillance of the elderly living alone can be more explicit than this. While public spaces are festooned with CCTV cameras, we expect our private home to remain private – yet the home of a frail elderly person can now be 'wired'. One or more family members go online to check, for example, that their elderly parent has gone to the bathroom this morning, opened the fridge door, or turned on the kettle. If such routines have not been performed, the relative contacts a designated neighbour to check on the old person. Some old people may welcome this surveillance, feeling it enables them to remain longer in their own home and possibly to die there. Others, though, may resent their daughter-in-law monitoring each time they visit the bathroom.

I have come across only one example of software that reverses the surveillance so that the housebound old person gets regular updates on how younger, fitter members of the family are doing. These family members upload pictures, music, text and other media depicting recent activity, displayed on a simple device on the housebound person's wall and accessed by a one-touch button. A short message such as 'Going to Sam's birthday party on Thursday' reminds the elderly person of her grandchild's upcoming birthday; she then uses old media – the telephone – to ask a neighbour to buy a card or a present, bring it to the house for her to sign, and then post it.

The remains

Migrant families have to decide where to bury the body, or what to do with cremated remains. The three main options are to conduct the funeral and bury in the 'host' country, in the 'home' country, or both – readily achieved with cremation where the ashes can be divided. Some researchers argue that the decision to bury in the 'host' country indicates integration. Hunter's (2016) interviews with Middle Eastern Christians living in Sweden, Denmark and Britain, however, indicate that it is not always this simple. Hunter summarises the many potential considerations influencing where to bury. Practical considerations include the difficulty of organising the funeral in one country compared to the other, security implications of taking the body home, and finance: the cost of air-freighting the body home may be mitigated by a cheaper and less bureaucratic funeral there. Territorial considerations include personal feelings about landscape; also the larger the person's ethnic community in the host country the more likely they are to be buried there. Religious considerations include standing up for one's religion in a place where it is under threat. And family considerations include the desire to rest with other family members, or to provide a founding grave as a focus for future generations, as illustrated by a young Iraqi: 'My grandmother…lived in Germany, but because she has three daughters here in Denmark she actually chose to be buried in Denmark' (Hunter, 2016, 186). Where to bury can cause conflict, not least between the deceased's spouse and family of origin. Migrants may live in two worlds, but how those worlds are constructed, and hence what is a good death or the best burial place, may be contested (Cohen and Odhiambo, 1992; van der Pijl, 2016).

Throughout history, people have not always died where they or their survivors wish them to be buried. As well as the desire to be buried 'back home', people may also want to be buried *away* from home. In nineteenth-century Britain, some of the new out-of-town cemeteries became highly fashionable, with special trains taking the urban dead and their mourners to these Elysian ex-urban fields. In the twenty-first century, some Britons choose a natural burial ground that is by no means the nearest but suits their taste or symbolises a personal connection. A neighbour of mine chose for her train-loving husband a natural burial ground which was a two-hour drive away as it is adjacent to a private steam railway line; visits to his grave are accompanied by both birdsong and the occasional whistle from a passing train. Some people are thus *more* mobile in death than they were in life.

Though burial is decidedly material and can take place in only one geographical location, graves are increasingly enmeshed in digital networks. Digitising cemetery records and putting them online enables genealogists the other side of the world to find where their ancestors are buried. Though QR codes embedded on gravestones may prove a short-lived fad, more flexible technologies will enable visitors to the grave to use their smart phone to call up pictures and a biography of the deceased; in turn, visitors may disseminate selfies of themselves at the graveside to relatives around the world or upload them to the deceased's memorial page. As in the rest of life so at the graveside, physical and virtual activity are inseparable for increasing numbers of people (Christensen and Sandvick, 2016).

Digital legacy

Only one person can inherit a material item. This can be contentious within families when, for example, one of the deceased's children inherits an item that has personal meaning to another child, or when one child receives the lion's share of the estate. Increasingly, what people now leave behind is digital – emails, social media accounts, picture collections, music collections – enabling inheritance of the same material by multiple friends and family members, irrespective of where in the world they are, and irrespective of whether they are at home or on the move.

At the same time, though, few people carefully read the service provider's fine print or think through how to make their digital property available, or not available, after their death. Most of those who use work email for personal messages have not thought whether their employer will grant the family access to these emails should they die. Some digital music collections are not owned outright but leased to the purchaser for his or her lifetime; informing the provider of the lessee's death may cause the collection instantly to vanish. Changing passwords regularly and keeping them secret, as we are regularly urged to do, risks rendering digital property inaccessible after death. Some companies now offer a digital 'safe' where passwords can be stored until the user's death, at which time they can be accessed by a nominated survivor; but this service is not free, nor is there any guarantee the 'safe' company or its technology will outlive the possibly youthful customer. The digital industry's death-denying reliance on secret passwords needs re-thinking.

Mourning

Social media not only enable contact with and between geographically distant mourners, but also re-insert as mourners those who are *socially* distant from the deceased.

As already noted, death has moved from the province of childhood to that of old age. Before this demographic transition, the deceased was likely to have been a child or a parent with young children. The main mourners therefore lived together, most likely in a one-room dwelling, so the loss was a shared experience – though, given individual variations in how people grieve (Doka and Martin, 2002), being forced together with others who might be grieving differently could lead to conflict or to a norm to keep one's grief to oneself and hence loneliness (Evans et al, 2016). The household might be located in a village of 100–200 souls who would hear of the death; though not main mourners, the village had lost a member, so everyone shared in mourning, to a greater or lesser degree.

Today, however, the main mourners have long since grown up and set up their own households, so are geographically separated. Thus, for example, when my father died age 90, the main mourners were my mother living in the house to which she and my father had retired; my brother and his family, living 50 miles east; and myself, 50 miles south. With the separation of home and work, working-age mourners daily go to a workplace where colleagues have probably never met the deceased. Colleagues may offer condolences, 'I'm sorry to hear about your father', but – having never met him – they are not themselves sorry he has died but sorry about my loss. They are positioned, not like villagers of old as co-mourners, but as supporters. Hence today there is much talk of how to 'support' the bereaved. Non-family mourners, such as the deceased's friends, colleagues, ex-colleagues, fellow members of church or sports club, are also more or less separated from each other. Though fellow sports club members may know each other, and likewise neighbours, the sports club members may not know the neighbours or the friends. The social network of mourners – primary and secondary – is fragmented; mourners are isolated from one another. It is hardly surprising that twentieth-century grief became, in many countries, internal, private.

Social media such as Facebook bring back into contact hitherto separate bits of a person's social network: in death as in life, if close family, friends, colleagues and sports club members are my Facebook friends, they all get to see what each other is posting. This brings hitherto fragmented mini-networks of mourners back into one online network – excepting perhaps a few older family members who are not on Facebook. The social network of mourners begins to resemble that of the pre-industrial village (Walter, 2015).

As in the pre-industrial village, this also opens the door to conflict. Especially in a United States split between secular people and devout believers, condolence posts asserting or implicitly denying an afterlife may offend some readers. Other forms of conflict become possible, or at least more visible. Pressure to be seen to join the virtual mourning can cause some who are not close to, or even dislike, the deceased to express what others may feel are crocodile tears. Conflict can also erupt over the control of social mourning. When a young adult dies, most of those posting condolences and memories online are other young adults; the deceased's grief-stricken parent, if not already their child's Facebook friend, will not be able to become their friend post-mortem. Parents who *can* access the online community of mourning may be comforted by the many posts; or they may be distressed by the levity of posts that fail to mirror the parent's intense grief. Should they then close down the page to protect themselves, but in the process deny lesser mourners the opportunity to share their feelings?

Social media mourning is no better or worse than the lonely privacy of twentieth-century mourning or the intrusive gossip of village mourning. It is what it is – offering both new possibilities and new problems. As with every aspect of death, each era creates new opportunities and challenges. With many millions of Facebook users now having died, Facebook as a company regularly reviews its memorialisation policy; aware of the issues that can arise after a user's death, the company engages in research to introduce more 'bereavement-friendly' features (Brubaker and Callison-Burch, 2016).

Connecting to the dead

Social and digital media have an uncanny ability to link mourners not only with one another but also with the dead. Online the dead can seem closer.

Social media post-mortem posts are often not *about* the dead, but addressed *to* them. People have probably spoken to the dead since time immemorial but in western societies in the twentieth century this was typically private: under your breath, or at the graveside when nobody else was around. But online, posts to the dead are not only common, they are – on some sites – expected: 'Happy birthday!' 'There's been a really bright star in the sky lately and I know it's you' (Kasket, 2012). Posting to/about the dead can indicate social distinction or assumed familiarity. Thus on Ministry of Defence memorial sites to British soldiers killed in Afghanistan, officers refer to the dead in the third person ('James was a star player in his platoon's football team'), while his mates use the second person ('Jimmie, our squad will never be the same without you').

Online, there are surprising mentions of heaven in otherwise secular posts – 'Hope you're having fun playing with the angels in heaven!' Posting messages to the deceased implies the deceased exists in some place, and in a post-Christian society that place is most readily described as heaven (Jakoby and Reiser, 2013). Also noticeable is the tendency of some mourners to address the deceased as an angel (Walter, 2016a). Angels, unlike souls, have wings, traversing the boundary between heaven and earth, between life and death; and unlike souls locked up in heaven, angels can read social media posts. Thus technological development affords a new space for, if not creedal faith, then spiritual discourse.

Whereas most social media are designed for life but may get used as communication tools in mourning when users die, other sites are designed specifically for communication after a death. Paula Kiel found three kinds at the time of her research (2016). First are sites that offer administrative closure – making arrangements for online assets, deleting specific accounts or folders, forwarding emails, automatic replies, and so on. All the sites of this kind she identified were active; none had closed. Second are sites offering social and emotional closure in which the deceased leaves family and friends a last message or sends a number of pre-written emails up to a year after the death. Only about half these sites were still active, possibly indicating people's ambivalence at arranging to send messages that some recipients might feel uncanny. Third are sites offering long-term communication from the dead, for example using AI (artificial intelligence) to analyse a customer's texts so that, after his or her death, the AI software can generate and send texts of a kind and in a language that s/he might have sent. Several of these sites have now ceased operation, possibly indicating AI's current limits.

In other words, bespoke post-mortem sites are most likely to be commercially sustainable if they offer simple administrative functions. Offering to sustain ongoing communication with the dead is more risky – these sites' highly skilled designers have not yet achieved the cosy familiarity with the dead that has been readily achieved by millions of Facebook users. But the technology is constantly evolving, so who knows how much closer digital media will bring the dead to the living.

Question

Most people adapt technologies with which they are familiar (such as email, Facebook, WhatsApp) to the circumstances of dying or grieving, rather than buy bespoke products. How have you or your family used digital or social media at end of life? Discuss any practical or ethical issues involved.

Note

[1]   My thanks to Renske Visser for alerting me to the issues raised in this paragraph.

NINE

Pervasive death

While the death awareness movement inveighs against death denial and taboos (Chapters One and Two), social scientists more often highlight death's absence from everyday life. Death has become medicalised and professionalised, 'sequestered' from mainstream society, leaving many citizens de-skilled and unfamiliar with death. Since the early 2000s, however, this sociological picture has become more nuanced, even challenged, by researchers identifying a new presence of death and the dead, if often a paradoxical 'absent presence' (Howarth, 2000). This chapter asks if, and if so to what extent, a twentieth-century separation of death from everyday life in western societies is mutating into a pervasive presence, a mutation involving both ideas and institutions. We might term this a shift in frameworks, a paradigm shift, or a shift in what historian Philippe Ariès (1981) called *mentalité*.

To give an example. Chapter One noted that witnessing the death of a sibling or parent is, thankfully, no longer a normal part of childhood – though this means many grow up as though humans do not die. Others have worried that adults try to protect children from death and mourning, for example by avoiding the subject or keeping them away from funerals. But consider what we found in Chapter Eight: on social media such as Facebook, it has become common for young people to post messages about, or to, acquaintances who have died.

Music and pictures as well as text are shared. In the twenty-first century, though many still get through childhood without experiencing a family member's death, it is impossible to get through childhood without knowing that not only celebrities but also ordinary people – friends, acquaintances and friends of friends – die. This change has occurred independent of the death awareness movement, and without any sense of a taboo being broken. Young people are not responding to incitements to talk about death; they are just using, often with considerable creativity, the affordances of social media. Thus the dead gain a presence online, and mortality gains a presence in the lives of young people.

This chapter is about death's re-emerging presence. This may – but equally may not – entail the breaking of taboos or an increase of conversation (Chapter Two). Talk gives death and the dead a presence, but it is not the only way to render death present. Jacobsen (2016) considers western societies to be moving away from 'forbidden death' to 'spectacular death' in which death, dying and mourning increasingly become spectacles. Though there are similarities in the trends we each identify, the new pervasive death this chapter discusses is more ordinary than spectacular.

Separated death

Western modernity separated death from life, so death became largely invisible. The *dying* were removed to a hospital, nursing home or other institution, even if many of the preceding months had been spent in the person's own home (which could mean a care home or other kind of supported living). From the nineteenth century, fewer *dead bodies* were buried in the churchyard through which villagers regularly walked to worship; increasing numbers were taken to an out of town cemetery or (in the twentieth century) crematorium. Bodies thus moved from the community's heart to its periphery. *Mourners'* experience of separation and invisibility has been a bit more complex. Nineteenth-century mourners were easily identifiable by their clothing – mourning dress for women, a black armband for men – and upper-class female mourners were excluded from social activity for a specified time. Twentieth-century mourners who abandoned signs of mourning on their apparel were no longer marked out and became invisible – economic, social and political life could proceed without embarrassing reminders that some of those present were bereaved. Twentieth-century mourners were enjoined to let go of the dead, to separate from them, so that they could get on with life unencumbered by grief and by the dead – though as Chapter Seven showed, romanticism taught that love is eternal and transcends the grave. Twentieth-century *souls* were most often seen as having gone to heaven where, cut off from this world, they could enjoy the company of pre-deceased family members. Catholics, however, continued to pray to and for the dead, while a surprising number of bereaved people consult mediums to contact the dead and find out if they are okay (Hazelgrove, 2000).

In sum, western Protestant modernity kept death and the dying at its margins, rendered mourners invisible, and left the soul to itself. Though there have been counter trends, the dominant narrative was of separation. What drove this? Institutional explanations point to the medicalisation of life, concerns about hygiene, religious factors, or capitalism's need to minimise anything that might cause workers to take time off. Anthony Giddens' explanation is at a higher level of abstraction (1991, 156): 'The ontological security which modernity has purchased, on the level of day-to-day routines, depends on an institutional exclusion of social life from the fundamental existential issues which raise central moral dilemmas.' As well as death, Giddens' troublesome, excluded issues include madness, criminality, sickness, sexuality and nature. Rather than critically evaluate such diverse explanations, I want now to consider whether separation may be becoming a thing of the past.

Pervasive death

From movies to soap operas to news media, death is beloved by the mass media (McIlwain, 2005). But media deaths – often violent, youthful, tragic, or of celebrities or disaster victims (these latter often in the global

South) – do not represent the kinds of death western audiences are likely to encounter personally; it is therefore questionable that media portrayals of death seriously challenge death's sequestration, though there are exceptions (Walter, 2009). More significant, perhaps, are social media. Pervasive mobile social media enable social interaction any place, any time – not only between mourners but also with the dead. The social media dead may be celebrities, but may just as easily be your grandmother or my friend's friend. Social media return death and loss to centre stage.

Chapter Seven described the notion of continuing bonds which re-valorises the romantic idea of eternal love that crosses the grave. By continuing bonds, the living move on with the dead, not without, them. This is expressed in online posts depicting the dead not as souls cut off in heaven but as angels travelling back and forth to earth, protecting the living. And as Chapter Six showed, the idea of the dead being disposed of is mutating – at least in British funeral industry discourse – into the dead being dispersed into the physical environments which sustain the living. Thus the personality, the spirit and the bodies of the dead all pervade everyday life.

Chapter Two showed how moral entrepreneurs are challenging 'the death taboo', urging everyone to talk about death. They portray a death-denying life as a life half lived; to live fully, death must be embraced. Starting in the 1970s, doctors – at least in individualistic countries that privilege personal autonomy (Chapter Three) – have come routinely to inform patients if their cancer is terminal, though communicating terminal prognosis with other diseases is less common. More recently, compassionate community initiatives around the world aim to return dying as well as death to the community (Chapter Four).

For the time being, however, the dying remain as segregated as ever. With the ageing of dying, increasing numbers of those on the last lap reside in care homes, while some with cognitive, mobility, hearing or sight impairments find themselves progressively isolated in their own home. And despite efforts to enable more people to die at home, most still draw their last breath in an institution. Aiming to counter isolation and stigmatisation, London's iconic St Christopher's Hospice, following the earlier example of the London Lighthouse for people with AIDS, has opened up a central café space where visitors do not immediately know if they are talking to other visitors, to staff or to people who are dying; yet the latter stages of dying continue to take place much less visibly, in side rooms. The deathbed is unlikely ever again to become the very public place Ariès (1981) depicts it as once having been. So, just as the separation of death from life was never total, so its new pervasiveness is far from total.

Nevertheless, something is going on. What might be driving it?

Drivers

So far, this book has suggested several drivers, such as the affordances of social media, a 200-year-old romantic sensibility about love, and a more recent ecological understanding that waste matter always remains in some form within the environment. It may also reflect what Linda Woodhead (2012) calls the 'de-reformation' of religion: 'Everyday, lived religion is thriving and evolving, while hierarchical, institutionalised, dogmatic forms of religion are marginalised. Religion has returned to the core business of sustaining everyday life, supporting relations with the living and the dead, and managing misfortune.' With the formal Protestant ban on relationships with the dead dissolving, it becomes easier to acknowledge continuing bonds with the dead, to creatively appropriate angels in the new online language of mourning, and for the funeral industry to offer spiritual comfort through the dead becoming part of the earth's ecosystem.

The blurring of the life/death, living/dead boundary may be part of a much broader cultural dissolution of boundaries that were central to modernity: male/female, gay/straight, human/animal (Howarth, 2000). This blurring and dissolving of categories might possibly be understood in terms of anthropological analysis of grid and group (Douglas, 1970); millennial dissolving of the bounded western individual (Smith, 2012); de-differentiation of institutions as production-oriented societies become consumer-driven societies (Davie, 2007); or replacement of Foucault's disciplinary society by

Deleuze's (1992) society of control. I simply mention these as possible lines of analysis.

Who is promoting the new paradigm of the pervasive dead? In this book and elsewhere (Walter, 1994), I have suggested the significance of female baby-boomer members of the expressive professions. Certainly their presence is evident in the death awareness movement in terms of leadership, writing, speaking at and attending movement meetings, and hands-on care of the dying and bereaved. They include doctors, nurses, counsellors, psychotherapists and social entrepreneurs within the funeral industry. The two high priestesses who inspired baby-boomer death reform were both doctors, Cicely Saunders disseminating her innovative care of the dying through internships at St Christopher's Hospice, and Elisabeth Kübler-Ross through international book publishing.

Cann's (2014) analysis of new everyday forms of memorialisation in the USA – located not in the cemetery but on tattoos, tee-shirts, car decals and social media – is that they are not driven by professionals but are grassroots. Innovations in memorialisation are made by those, often Hispanic, whose grief – and to some extent their life – has been marginalised and who wish to claim the status of mourner. And this certainly fits my understanding of mourning by non-family on social media.

These explanations may be reconciled. a) There is a top-down death awareness movement. Sometimes death awareness is formally mandated from above as in end of life care policies, the UK's *Dying Matters Coalition*, some compassionate community initiatives and the many medical schools that train their students how to communicate about dying. Sometimes the passion for death awareness is found in individual counsellors, nurses or entrepreneurs who join together through less formal means such as the **home death** movement, the natural death movement, and **doula** (death midwife) training. All these are dominated by baby-boomer members of the expressive professions. b) At the same time there are bottom-up innovations of the kind Cann discusses which are happening entirely independently of the death awareness movement and its incitements to talk. People just post stuff on social media, get a memorial tattoo, or buy a memorial decal for their car's rear window, without any sense of being part of a movement or breaking so-called taboos. But the effects of such actions are similar: they bring death, dying, mourning and the dead out of the shadows into the warp and woof of everyday life.

Not everybody welcomes this, however…

Counter trends

I have already noted that the deathbed remains sequestrated from everyday life. There are some areas where separation of the dead is increasing, rather than dissolving. The twenty-first century has witnessed a new squeamishness, at least in a small but influential minority, at viewing human remains in museums (Jenkins, 2010). Many western museums now place human remains in specially marked display areas, with signs warning visitors before they enter so that they can make an informed choice whether or not the view the remains. The UK Ministry of Justice ruled in 2008 that archaeologists who unearth human bones, however ancient, should after any scientific analysis re-bury them; following protests, the Ministry subsequently relaxed the regulations so it is now again possible for bones to be placed in museums (Parker Pearson et al, 2013).

Culture also influences what aspects of death may or may not be seen. Thus in English culture, viewing of the body in the funeral parlour is private, with a handful of family members, or no-one at all, viewing. In the USA, by contrast, viewing of the embalmed body is a community affair to which all are welcome (Harper, 2010). Indeed, inviting the community into the funeral parlour to appreciate the care with which the deceased is cared for and displayed is central to the American funeral director's business model. This does not, however, mean that Americans are more comfortable with dead bodies in public places. Whereas English people are used to seeing glass-sided hearses passing by in their local high street, American hearses hide their contents; passers-by know it is a hearse, but the casket is not visible. What this comparison shows is that death is neither entirely pervasive nor entirely sequestrated, neither completely visible nor completely invisible; rather, *how* it becomes partly visible, *how* elements come to pervade everyday life, depends on culture. Introducing glass-sided hearses to Americans, or public viewing to the English, would likely fail.

How many twenty-first century people will embrace the new paradigm of pervasive death, and in what ways, or how they will combine it with the old paradigm of separation, only time will tell. Many people may continue to exercise their right to live without thought of death; many may prefer to live without memories of the dead, at least some of the time. They may prefer to walk their dog in the local park without every bench they pass bearing a memorial plaque to a dead person; to go shopping without encountering *memento mori* in the form of roadside shrines; to go online without encountering memorial posts. To quote the Peanuts cartoon:

'Some day, we will all die, Snoopy!'
'True, but on all other days we will not.'

End of life care policies and practices, memorialisation policies in local communities and in social media, employers' compassionate leave policies, health promotion messages, and the death awareness movement all need to strike a balance between Peanuts' two simple truths.

References

Abel, J, Bowra, J, Walter, T et al, 2011, Compassionate community networks: Supporting home dying, *BMJ Supportive and Palliative Care* 2, 129–33

Agamben, G, 1998, *Homo sacer: Sovereign power and bare life*, Stanford, CA: Stanford University Press

Aldridge, MD, Kelley, AS, 2015, The myth regarding the high cost of end-of-life care, *American Journal of Public Health* 105, 2411–15

Ariès, P, 1981, *The hour of our death*, London: Allen Lane

Armstrong, D, 1987, Silence and truth in death and dying, *Social Science and Medicine* 24, 651–7

Arney, WR, Bergen, BJ, 1984, *Medicine and the management of living*, Chicago, IL: University of Chicago Press

Aveline-Dubach, N, 2012, *Invisible population: The place of the dead in East Asian megacities*, Lanham, MD: Lexington Books

Baeke, G, Wils, JP, Broeckaert, B, 2011, We are (not) the master of our body: Elderly Jewish women's attitudes towards euthanasia and assisted suicide, *Ethnicity and Health* 16, 259–78

Bauman, Z, 1992, *Mortality, immortality and other life strategies*, Cambridge: Polity

Bayatrizi, Z, Tehrani RT, 2017, The objective life of death in Tehran: A vanishing presence, *Mortality* 22, 15–32

Becker, E, 1973, *The denial of death*, New York: Free Press

Berger, P, 1969, *The social reality of religion*, London: Faber

Bernstein, A, 2006, *Modern passings: Death rites, politics, and social change in Imperial Japan*, Honolulu, HI: University of Hawai'i Press

Blauner, R, 1966, Death and social structure, *Psychiatry* 29, 378–94

Bloch, M, 1971, *Placing the dead: Tombs, ancestral villages and kinship organisation in Madagascar*, London and New York: Seminar Press

Bonanno, GA, 2004, Loss, trauma, and human resilience: Have we underestimated the human capacity to thrive after extremely aversive events?, *American Psychologist* 59, 20–8

Borgstrom, E, Walter, T, 2015, Choice and compassion at the end of life: A critical analysis of recent English policy discourse, *Social Science and Medicine* 136–7, 99–105

Bowlby, J, 1961, Processes of mourning, *The International Journal of Psychoanalysis* 42, 317–40

Boyle, G, Warren, L, 2017, Showing how they feel: The emotional reflexivity of people with dementia, *Families, Relationships and Societies* 6, 3–19

Bramley, L, 2016, One day at a time: Living with frailty: implications for the practice of advance care planning, Nottingham: University of Nottingham, PhD thesis. http://eprints.nottingham. ac.uk/33400/7/Final%20post%20viva%20uploaded%20Bramley.pd

Bravo, V, 2017, Coping with dying and deaths at home: How undocumented migrants in the United States experience the process of transnational grieving, *Mortality* 22, 33–44

Brubaker, JR, Callison-Burch, V, 2016, Legacy contact: Designing and implementing post-mortem stewardship at Facebook, *Proceedings of CHI 2016*, San Jose, CA

Brubaker, JR, Hayes, GR, Dourish, P, 2013, Beyond the grave: Facebook as a site for the expansion of death and mourning, *The Information Society* 29, 152–63

Butler, RN, 1963, The life review: An interpretation of reminiscence in the aged, *Psychiatry* 26, 65–76

Campbell, C, 1987, *The romantic ethic and the spirit of modern consumerism*, Oxford: Blackwell

Cann, CK, 2014, *Virtual afterlives: Grieving the dead in the twenty-first century,* Lexington, KY: University Press of Kentucky

Caswell, G, O'Connor, M, 2015, Agency in the context of social death: Dying alone at home, *Contemporary Social Science* 10, 249–61

Christensen, DR, Sandvick, K, 2016, Grief to everyday life: Bereaved parents' negotiations of presence across media, in K Sandvik, AM Thorhauge, B Valtysson (eds) *The media and the mundane: Communication across media in everyday life*, pp 105–18, Gothenburg: Nordicom

Clark, D, 1999, 'Total pain', disciplinary power and the body in the work of Cicely Saunders, 1958–1967, *Social Science and Medicine* 49, 727–36

Clark, D, Inbadas, H, Colburn, D et al, 2017, Interventions at the end of life: A taxonomy for 'overlapping consensus', *Wellcome Open Research* 2. https://wellcomeopenresearch.org/articles/2-7/v1

Cohen, DW, Odhiambo, ESA, 1992, *Burying SM: The politics of knowledge and the sociology of power in Africa*, Nairobi: East African Educational Publishers

Cohen, RL, 2011, Time, space and touch at work: Body work and labour process (re)organisation, *Sociology of Health and Illness* 33, 189–205

Coleman, P, Ivani-Chalian, C, Robinson, M, 2015, *Self and meaning in the lives of older people*, Cambridge: Cambridge University Press

Conway, S, 2011, *Governing death and loss: Empowerment, involvement and participation*, Oxford: Oxford University Press

Cook, G, Walter, T, 2005, Rewritten rites: Language and social relations in traditional and contemporary funerals, *Discourse and Society* 16, 365–91

Coombs, S, 2014, Death wears a T-shirt – listening to young people talk about death, *Mortality* 19, 284–302

Corden, A, Hirst, M, 2013, Financial constituents of family bereavement, *Family Science* 4, 59–65

Currier, JM, Neimeyer, R, Berman, JS, 2008, The effectiveness of psychotherapeutic interventions for the bereaved: A comprehensive quantitative review, *Psychological Bulletin* 134, 648–61

Danely J, 2014, *Aging and loss: Mourning and maturity in contemporary Japan*, New Brunswick, NJ: Rutgers University Press

Danforth, L, 1982, *The death rituals of Rural Greece,* Princeton, NJ: Princeton University Press

Davie, G, 2007, *The sociology of religion*, London: Sage

Davies, D, 2015, *Mors Britannica: Lifestyle and death-style in Britain today*, Oxford: Oxford University Press

Davies, D, Rumble H, 2012, *Natural burial: Traditional–secular spiritualities and funeral innovation*, London: Continuum

DEFRA (Department for Environment Food and Rural Affairs), 2003, *Mercury emissions from crematoria*, London: DEFRA

Deleuze, G, 1992, Postscript on the Societies of Control, *October* 59, 3–7

Doi, T, 1981, *The anatomy of dependence*, Tokyo: Kodansha International

Doka, KJ, 1989, *Disenfranchised grief: Recognizing hidden sorrow*, Lanham, MD: Lexington Books

Doka, KJ, Martin, TL, 2002, How we grieve: Culture, class, and gender, in KJ Doka (ed) *Disenfranchised grief: New directions, challenges, and strategies for practice*, pp 337–47, Champaign, IL: Research Press

Dorling, D, 2013, *Unequal health: The scandal of our times*, Bristol: Policy Press

Douglas, M, 1966, *Purity and danger: An analysis of concepts of pollution and taboo*, London: Routledge and Kegan Paul

Douglas, M, 1970, *Natural symbols: Explorations in cosmology*, New York: Pantheon

Draper, JW, 1967, *The funeral elegy and the rise of English Romanticism*, London: Frank Cass

du Boulay, S, 1984, *Cicely Saunders*, London: Hodder

Durkheim, E, 1915, *The elementary forms of the religious life*, London: Unwin

EIU (Economist Intelligence Unit), 2015, *The 2015 Quality of Death Index: Ranking palliative care across the world*, London: EIU

Eisenbruch, M, 1984, Cross-cultural aspects of bereavement, *Culture, Medicine and Psychiatry* 8, 283–309, 315–47

Elias, N, 1985, *The loneliness of the dying*, Oxford: Blackwell

Evans, R, Ribbens McCarthy, J, Bowlby, S et al, 2016, Responses to death, care and family relations in urban Senegal, *Human Geography Research Cluster,* Reading: University of Reading. http://blogs. reading.ac.uk/deathinthefamilyinsenegal/files/2017/03/Evans-et-al-2016-Report-1.pdf

Field, D, 1996, Awareness and modern dying, *Mortality* 1, 255–65

Fine, B, 2010, *Theories of social capital: Researchers behaving badly,* London: Pluto

Firth, S, 1997, *Dying, death and bereavement in a British Hindu community,* Leuven: Peeters

Fitzpatrick, R, Chandola, T, 2000, Health, in AH Halsey, J Webb (eds) *Twentieth-century British social trends,* pp 94–127, Basingstoke: Macmillan

Fong, J, 2017, *The death café movement: Exploring the horizons of mortality,* New York: Palgrave Macmillan

Foote, C, Frank, AW, 1999, Foucault and therapy: The discipline of grief, in A Chambon, A Irving, L Epstein (eds) *Reading Foucault for social work,* pp 157–87, New York: Columbia University Press

Foster, L, Woodthorpe, K, 2013, What cost the price of a good send off? The challenges for British state funeral policy, *Journal of Poverty and Social Justice* 21, 77–89

Foucault, M, 1973, *The birth of the clinic: An archaeology of medical perception,* London: Tavistock

Francis, D, Kellaher, L, Neophytou, G, 2005, *The secret cemetery,* Oxford: Berg

Francis, R, 2013, *The Mid Staffordshire NHS Foundation Trust public inquiry: Final report,* London: The Stationery Office

Freud, S, 1917, Mourning and melancholia, in S Freud (ed) *On metapsychology,* pp 251–67, London: Pelican, 1984

Friedman, L, 2014, A burning question: The climate impact of 7 million funeral pyres in India and Nepal, *E&E News,* 27 January

Furedi, F, 2004, *Therapy culture: Cultivating vulnerability in an uncertain age,* London: Routledge

Garces-Foley, K, Holcomb, JS, 2005, Contemporary American funerals: Personalizing tradition, in K Garces-Foley (ed) *Death and religion in a changing world*, pp 207–27, Armonk, NY: ME Sharpe

Gardner, PJ, 2011, Natural neighborhood networks: Important social networks in the lives of older adults aging in place, *Journal of Aging Studies* 25, 263–71

Giddens, A, 1991, *Modernity and self-identity: Self and society in the late modern age*, Cambridge: Polity

Gilleard, C, Higgs, P, 2010, Aging without agency: Theorizing the fourth age, *Aging and Mental Health* 14, 121–8

Gilligan, C, 1982, *In a different voice: Psychological theory and women's development*, Cambridge, MA: Harvard University Press

Gittings, C, 1984, *Death, burial and the individual in early modern England*, London: Croom Helm

GMC (General Medical Council), 2010, *Treatment and care towards the end of life: Good practice in decision making*, London: GMC

Goffman, E, 1961, *Asylums*, Garden City: Anchor

Gorer, G, 1965, *Death, grief and mourning in contemporary Britain*, London: Cresset

Gunaratnam, Y, 2013, *Death and the migrant: Bodies, borders and care*, London: Bloomsbury

Halpern, SD, 2015, Toward evidence-based end-of-life care, *New England Journal of Medicine* 373, 2001–03

Harper, S, 2010, Behind closed doors? Corpses and mourners in American and English funeral premises, in J Hockey, C Komaromy, K Woodthorpe (eds) *The matter of death: Space, place and materiality*, pp 100–16, Basingstoke: Palgrave MacMillan

Hazelgrove, J, 2000, *Spiritualism and British society between the wars*, Manchester: Manchester University Press

Heimerl, K, Wegleitner, K, 2013, Organizational and health system change through participatory research, in J Hockley, K Froggatt, K Heimerl (eds) *Participatory research in palliative care*, pp 27–39, Oxford: Oxford University Press

Hertz, R, 1907, A contribution to the study of the collective representation of death, *Death and the right hand*, pp 27–86, London: Cohen and West,1960

Hetherington, K, 2004, Second-handedness: Consumption, disposal and absent presence, *Environment and Planning D: Society and Space* 22, 157–73

Hockey, J, Kellaher, L, Prendergast, D, 2007, Sustaining kinship: Ritualization and the disposal of human ashes in the United Kingdom, in M Mitchell (ed) *Remember me*, pp 33–50, London: Routledge

Holst-Warhaft, G, 2000, *The cue for passion: Grief and its political uses*, Cambridge, MA: Harvard University Press

Horsfall, D, Noonan, K, Leonard, R, 2011, *Bringing our dying home: Creating community at the end of life*, Sydney: University of Western Sydney

Horsfall, D, Leonard, R, Noonan, K et al, 2013, Working together – apart: Exploring the relationships between formal and informal care networks for people dying at home, *Progress in Palliative Care* 21, 331–36

Howarth, G, 1996, *Last rites: The work of the modern funeral director*, Amityville, NY: Baywood

Howarth, G, 2000, Dismantling the boundaries between life and death, *Mortality* 5, 127–38

Hughes, P, Turton, P, Hopper, E et al, 2002, Assessment of guidelines for good practice in psychosocial care of mothers after stillbirth: A cohort study, *Lancet* 360, 114–18

Hunter, A, 2016, Staking a claim to land, faith and family: Burial location preferences of Middle Eastern Christian migrants, *Journal of Intercultural Studies* 37, 179–94

Illich, I, 1975, *Medical nemesis: The expropriation of health*, London: Calder and Boyars

Inglehart R, 1981, Post-materialism in an environment of insecurity, *American Political Science Review* 75, 880–900

Jacobsen, MH, 2016, 'Spectacular death': Proposing a new fifth phase to Philippe Ariès's admirable history of death, *Humanities* 5, 19

Jakoby, NR, Reiser, S, 2013, Grief 2.0. Exploring virtual cemeteries, in T Benski, E Fisher (eds) *Internet and emotions*, pp 65–79, London: Routledge

Jalland, P, 2010, *Death in war and peace: A history of loss and grief in England, 1914–1970*, Oxford: Oxford University Press

Jenkins, T, 2010, *Contesting human remains in museum collections: The crisis of cultural authority*, London: Routledge

Jindra, M, Noret, J, 2011, *Funerals in Africa: Explorations of a social phenomenon*, Oxford: Berghahn

Johnson, M, 2016, Spirituality, biographical review and biographical pain at the end of life in old age, in M Johnson, J Walker (eds) *Spiritual dimensions of ageing*, pp 198–214, Cambridge: Cambridge University Press

Jupp, P, 2006, *From dust to ashes: Cremation and the British way of death*, Basingstoke and New York: Palgrave Macmillan

Kamerman, J, 2002, Balancing the costs of enfranchising the disenfranchised griever, in KJ Doka (ed) *Disenfranchised grief: New directions, challenges, and strategies for practice*, pp 405–12, Champaign, IL: Research Press

Kaminer, H, Lavie, P, 1993, Sleep and dreams in well-adjusted and less adjusted Holocaust survivors, in M Stroebe, W Stroebe, R Hansson (eds) *Handbook of bereavement: Theory, research, and intervention*, pp 331–45, Cambridge: Cambridge University Press

Kasket, E, 2012, Continuing bonds in the age of social networking: Facebook as a modern-day medium, *Bereavement Care* 31, 62–9

Kaufman, S, 2005, *…And a time to die: How American hospitals shape the end of life*, Chicago, IL: University of Chicago Press

Kellehear, A, 1984, Are we a death-denying society? A sociological review, *Social Science and Medicine* 18, 713–23

Kellehear, A, 1996, *Experiences near death: Beyond medicine and religion*, Oxford: Oxford University Press

Kellehear, A, 1999, *Health promoting palliative care*, Oxford: Oxford University Press

Kellehear, A, 2005, *Compassionate cities*, London: Routledge

Kellehear, A, 2007, *A social history of dying*, Cambridge: Cambridge University Press

Kellehear, A, 2009, Dying old – and *preferably* alone? Agency, resistance and dissent at the end of life, *International Journal of Ageing and Later Life* 4, 5–21

Kellehear, A, 2014, *The inner life of the dying person*, New York: Columbia University Press

Kellehear, A, 2016, Current social trends and challenges for the dying person, in NR Jakoby, M Thönnes (eds) *Zur Soziologie des Sterbens*, pp 11–26, Berlin: Springer VS

Kiel, P, 2016, Online after death: Practices of (un)controlled presence, *Death, dying and bereavement and technologies in the 21C* conference, Sheffield, 2 December

Kitch, C, Hume, J, 2008, *Journalism in a culture of grief*, New York: Routledge

Kjaersgaard Markussen, A, 2013, Death and the state of Denmark: Believing, belonging and doing, in E Venbrux, T Quartier, C Venhorst, B Mathijssen (eds) *Changing European death ways*, pp 165–8, Münster: LIT Verlag

Klass, D, Heath, AO, 1997, Grief and abortion: Mizuko kuyo, the Japanese ritual resolution, *Omega* 34, 1–14

Klass, D, Silverman, PR, Nickman, SL, 1996, *Continuing bonds: New understandings of grief*, Bristol, PA: Taylor and Francis

Kretchmer, A, 2000, Mortuary rites for inanimate objects: The case of Hari Kuyō, *Japanese Journal of Religious Studies* 27, 379–404

Kubasak, MW, 1990, *Cremation and the funeral director: Successfully meeting the challenge*, Malibu: Avalon Press

Kübler-Ross, E, 1969, *On death and dying*, New York: Macmillan

Kumar, S, 2007, Kerala, India: A regional community-based palliative care model, *Journal of Pain and Symptom Management* 33, 623–27

LaFleur, W, 1992, *Liquid life: Abortion and Buddhism in Japan*, Princeton, NJ: Princeton University Press

Laquer, T, 2015, *The work of the dead: A cultural history of mortal remains*, Princeton, NJ: Princeton University Press

Lee, E, 2003, *Abortion, motherhood and mental health: Medicalizing reproduction in the United States and Great Britian*, New Brunswick, NJ: Transaction

Leonard, R, Horsfall, D, Noonan, K, 2013, Identifying changes in the support networks of end-of-life carers using social network analysis, *BMJ Supportive and Palliative Care* 3, 383–8, doi:10.1136/bmjspcare-2012000257

Lloyd, L, 2004, Mortality and morality: Ageing and the ethics of care, *Ageing and Society* 24, 235–56

Lloyd, L, Banerjee, A, Jacobsen, FF et al, 2014, It's a scandal! Comparing the causes and consequences of nursing home media scandals in five countries, *International Journal of Sociology and Social Policy* 34, 2–18

Lofland, L, 1978, *The craft of dying: The modern face of death*, Beverly Hills, CA: Sage

Lofland, L, 1985, The social shaping of emotion: The case of grief, *Symbolic Interaction* 8, 171–90

Loudon, JC, 1843, *On the laying out, planting, and managing of cemeteries and on the improvement of churchyards*, Redhill: Ivelet Books, 1981

Love, N, 2009, NH rejects dissolving bodies as cremation alternative, *Seacoastonline.com*. www.seacoastonline.com/article/20090304/NEWS/90304045

Lynn, J, Adamson, DM, 2003, *Living well at the end of life: Adapting health care to serious chronic illness in old age*, Santa Monica, CA: Rand

McDannell, C, Lang, B, 2001, *Heaven – a history*, New Haven, CT: Yale University Press

McIlwain, CD, 2005, *When death goes pop: Death, media and the remaking of community*, New York: Peter Lang

McKeown, T, 1979, *The role of medicine*, Oxford: Blackwell

McManus, R, Schafer, C, 2014, Final arrangements: Examining debt and distress, *Mortality* 19, 379–97

Marris, P, 1958, *Widows and their families*, London: Routledge

Martin, B, 1981, *A sociology of contemporary cultural change*, Oxford: Blackwell

Maruyama, TC, 1997, The Japanese pilgrimage: Not begun, *International Journal of Palliative Nursing* 3, 87–91

Mellor, P, Shilling, C, 1993, Modernity, self-identity and the sequestration of death, *Sociology* 27, 411–31

Mitford, J, 1963, *The American way of death*, London: Hutchinson

Mitscherlich, A, Mitscherlich, M, 1975, *The inability to mourn*, New York: Grove Press

Mol, A, 2008, *The logic of care: Health and the problem of patient choice*, London: Routledge

Moore, J, 2012, Being there: Technology at the end of life, in CJ Sofka, IN Cupit, KR Gilbert (eds) *Dying, death and grief in an online universe*, pp 78–86, New York: Springer

Norwood, F, 2009, *The maintenance of life: Preventing social death through euthanasia talk and end-of-life care – lessons from The Netherlands*, Durham, NC: Carolina Academic Press

Novack, DH, Plumer, R, Smith, RL, 1979, Changes in physician's attitudes toward telling the cancer patient, *Journal of the American Medical Association* 241, 897–900

Parker Pearson, M, Pitts, M, Sayer, D, 2013, Changes in policy for excavating human remains in England and Wales, in M Giesen (ed) *Curating human remains: Caring for the dead in the United Kingdom*, pp 147–58, Woodbridge: Boydell and Brewer

Parkes, CM, 2008, *Love and loss: The roots of grief and its complications*, London: Routledge

Parsons, T, Lidz, V, 1963, Death in American society: A brief working paper, *American Behavioral Scientist* 6, 61–5

Pavicevic, A, 2009, Death in a foreign land: Entering and exiting the Serbian emigrant's world, in U Brunnbauer (ed) *Transnational societies, transterritorial politics, and migrations in the (post)Yugoslav area 19th–21st century*, pp 235–48, Munich: R Oldenbourg Verlag

Perri 6, 1997, *Escaping poverty: From safety nets to networks of opportunity*, London: Demos

Pincus, L, 1976, *Death and the family*, London: Faber

Power, M, 1997, *The audit society*, Oxford: Oxford University Press

Prendergast, D, Hockey, J, Kellaher, L, 2006, Blowing in the wind? Identity, materiality, and the destinations of human ashes, *Journal of the Royal Anthropological Institute* 12, 881–98

Prothero, S, 2000, *Purified by fire: A history of cremation in America*, Berkeley, CA: University of California Press

Putnam, RD, 2000, *Bowling alone: The collapse and revival of American community*, New York: Simon and Schuster

Raudon, S, 2011, *Contemporary funerals and mourning practices: An investigation of five secular countries*, Auckland, NZ: Winston Churchill Memorial Trust

Reynolds, JJ, 2002, Disenfranchised grief and the politics of helping: Social policy and its clinical implications, in KJ Doka (ed) *Disenfranchised grief: New directions, challenges, and strategies for practice*, pp 351–87, Champaign, IL: Research Press

Richardson, R, 1989, *Death, dissection and the destitute*, London: Penguin

Robson, P, Walter, T, 2012–13, Hierarchies of loss: A critique of disenfranchised grief, *Omega* 66, 97–119

Rose, N, 1989, *Governing the soul: The shaping of the private self*, London: Routledge

Rosenblatt, P, Walsh, P, Jackson, D, (eds) 1976, *Grief and mourning in cross-cultural perspective*, Washington, DC: Human Relations Area Files Press

Rotar, M, 2015, Attitudes towards cremation in contemporary Romania, *Mortality* 20, 145–62

Rumble, H, Troyer, J, Walter, T et al, 2014, Disposal or dispersal? Environmentalism and final treatment of the British dead, *Mortality* 19, 243–60

Russ, AJ, 2005, Love's labor paid for: Gift and commodity at the threshold of death, *Cultural Anthropology* 20, 128–55

Sallnow, L, Richardson, H, Murray, S et al, 2016, The impact of a new public health approach to end-of-life care: A systematic review, *Palliative Medicine* 30, 200–11

Scheper-Hughes, N, 1992, *Death without weeping: The violence of everyday life in Brazil*, Berkeley, CA: University of California Press

Schut, H, Stroebe, M, 2005, Interventions to enhance adaptation to bereavement, *Journal of Palliatiive Medicine* 8, 140–7

Schut, H, Stroebe, M, van den Bout, J et al, 1997, Intervention for the bereaved: Gender differences in the efficacy of two counselling programmes, *British Journal of Clinical Psychology* 36, 63–72

Scourfield, P, 2012, Cartelization revisited and the lessons of Southern Cross, *Critical Social Policy* 32, 137–48

Seymour, J, Witherspoon, R, Gott, M et al, 2005, *End-of-life care: Promoting comfort, choice and well-being for older people*, Bristol: Policy Press

Silveira, MJ, Kim, SYH, Langa, KM, 2010, Advance directives and outcomes of surrogate decision making before death, *New England Journal of Medicine* 362, 1211–18, doi:10.1056/NEJMsa0907901

Sloane, DC, 1991, *The last great necessity: Cemeteries in American history*, Baltimore, MD: Johns Hopkins University Press

Smith, K, 2012, From dividual and individual selves to porour subjects, *Australian Journal of Anthropology* 23, 50–64

Stroebe, M, Gergen, MM, Gergen, KJ et al, 1992, Broken hearts or broken bonds: Love and death in historical perspective, *American Psychologist* 47, 1205–12

Stroebe, MS, Schut, H, 1999, The dual process model of coping with bereavement: Rationale and description, *Death Studies* 23, 197–224

Sudnow, D, 1967, *Passing on: The social organization of dying*, Englewood Cliffs, NJ: Prentice Hall

Taylor, L, 1983, *Mourning dress: A costume and social history*, London: Allen and Unwin

Thomas, H, 2010, Resomation®: The debate (Part 1), *Pharos International* 76, 4–8

Thomas, H, 2011, Resomation®: The debate (Part 2), *Pharos International* 77, 4–8

Torrie, M, 1987, *My years with CRUSE*, Richmond: CRUSE

Townsend, P, 1964, *The last refuge*, London: Routledge

Trajectory, 2016, *Losing a partner: The financial and practical consequences*, London: Royal London

Tronto, JC, 1994, *Moral boundaries: A political argument for an ethic of care*, London: Routledge

Tronto, JC, 2010, Creating caring institutions: Politics, plurality, and purpose, *Ethics and Social Welfare* 4, 158–71

Twigg, J, 2006, *The body in health and social care*, Basingstoke: Palgrave Macmillan

Ungerson, C, 1997, Social politics and the commodification of care, *Social Politics* 4, 362–81

Utriainen, T, 2010, Agents of de-differentiation: Women care-givers for the dying in Finland, *Journal of Contemporary Religion* 25, 437–51

van der Pijl, Y, 2016, Death in the family revisited: Ritual expression and controversy in a Creole transnational mortuary sphere, *Ethnography* 17, 147–67

van Heijst, A, 2011, *Professional loving care: An ethical view of the health care sector*, Leuven: Peeters

Verkerk, M, 1999, A care perspective on coercion and autonomy, *Bioethics* 13, 358–68

Verkerk, M, 2001, The care perspective and autonomy, *Medicine, Health Care and Philosophy* 4, 289–94

Visser, R, 2017, 'Doing death': Reflecting on the researcher's subjectivity and emotions, *Death Studies* 41, 6–13

Walsh, M, Wrigley, C, 2001, Womanpower: The transformation of the labour force in the UK and the USA since 1945, *Refresh* 30, 1–4

Walter, T, 1990, *Funerals and how to improve them*, Sevenoaks: Hodder and Stoughton

Walter, T, 1994, *The revival of death*, London: Routledge

Walter, T, 1996, *The eclipse of eternity: A sociology of the afterlife*, Basingstoke: Macmillan

Walter, T, 1999a, A death in our street, *Health and Place* 5, 119–24

Walter, T, 1999b, *On bereavement: The culture of grief*, Buckingham: Open University Press

Walter, T, 2005, Three ways to arrange a funeral: Mortuary variation in the modern west, *Mortality* 10, 173–92

Walter, T, 2009, Jade's dying body: The ultimate reality show, *Sociological Research Online* 14, 5, doi:10.5153/sro.2061

Walter, T, 2015, New mourners, old mourners: Online memorial culture as a chapter in the history of mourning, *New Review of Hypermedia and Multimedia* 21, 1–2, Special issue: Online memorial cultures, 10–24

Walter, T, 2016a, The dead who become angels: Bereavement and vernacular religion, *Omega* 73, 3–28

Walter, T, 2016b, Judgement, myth and hope in life-centred funerals, *Theology* 119, 4, 253–60

Walter, T, 2017, How the dead survive: Ancestor, immortality, memory, in MH Jacobsen (ed) *Postmortal society: Multidisciplinary perspectives on death, survivalism and immortality in contemporary culture*, Farnham: Ashgate

Walter, T, Hourizi, R, Moncur, W, Pitsillides, S, 2011–12, Does the internet change how we die and mourn?, *Omega* 64, 275–302

Weber, M, 1930, *The Protestant ethic and the spirit of capitalism*, London: Allen and Unwin

Wegleitner, K, Heimerl, K, Kellehear, A, 2015, *Compassionate communities: Case studies from Britain and Europe*, London: Routledge

Wenger, GC, 1991, A network typology, from theory to practice, *Journal of Aging Studies* 5, 147–62

West, K, 2008, How green is my funeral?, *Funeral Service Journal* 123, 104–8

Winzelberg, GS, Hanson, LJ, Tulsky, J, 2005, Beyond autonomy: Diversifying end of life decision approaches to serve patients and families, *Journal of the American Geriatric Society* 53, 1046–50

Woodhead, L, 2012, Mind, body and spirit: It's the de-reformation of religion, *Guardian,* 7 May

Worden, JW, 1983, *Grief counselling and grief therapy*, London: Routledge

Work and Pensions Select Committee, 2016, *Support for the bereaved*, London: House of Commons, www.publications.parliament.uk/pa/cm201516/cmselect/cmworpen/551/55102.htm

Wortman, C, Silver, R, 1989, The myths of coping with loss, *Journal of Consulting and Clinical Psychology* 57, 349–57

Yamazaki, H, 2008, *Rethinking good death: Insights from a case analysis of a Japanese medical comic*, Oxford: Uehiro–Carnegie–Oxford Conference on Medical Ethics, University of Oxford, 11–12 December

Young, M, Cullen, L, 1996, *A good death: Conversations with East Londoners*, London: Routledge

Zerubavel, E, 2003, *Time maps: Collective memory and the social shape of the past*, Chicago, IL: University of Chicago Press

Zuckerman, P, 2008, *Society without God: What the least religious nations can tell us about contentment*, New York: New York University Press

Index